The Death
of a Disease

The Death of a Disease

A History of the Eradication of Poliomyelitis

Bernard Seytre
Mary Shaffer

Rutgers University Press

New Brunswick, New Jersey, and London

Originally published as *Histoire de l'éradication de la poliomyélite,*
© Presses Universitaires de France, 2004.

Library of Congress Cataloging-in-Publication Data

Seytre, Bernard.
  [Histoire de l'éradication de la poliomyélite. English]
  The death of a disease : a history of the eradication of poliomyeli-
tis / Bernard Seytre and Mary Shaffer ; translated by Mary Shaffer.
    p. ; cm.
  Includes bibliographical references and index.
  ISBN–13: 978–0–8135–3676–7 (hardcover : alk. paper)
  ISBN–13: 978–0–8135–3677–4 (pbk. : alk. paper)
  1. Poliomyelitis—History. 2. Poliomyelitis vaccine—History.
[DNLM: 1. Poliomyelitis—prevention & control. 2. History, 20th
Century. 3. Vaccination—history.] I. Shaffer, Mary. II. Title.

RC180.9.S4913   2005
616. 8'25–dc22

                                                        2005002654

A British Cataloging-in-Publication record for this book is available
from the British Library.

Manufactured in the United States of America

Contents

Acknowledgments

The authors are indebted to the many individuals who helped us piece together the stories in this book. Several people gave a great deal of time to share their memories, experience, and knowledge; guide us in the right direction; and reread our manuscript. Each knows what we owe them.

Our sincere thanks go to Bruce Aylward, Luis Barreto, Steve Cochi, Michel Galy, Shawn Gilchrist, George Giummarra, Michel Gréco, Gary Hlady, Wai Ing, Shirley Johnson, Cécile Lalande, Christine Laouénan, Mark Lievonen, Lucile Margaine, Bernard Montagnon, Pierre Morgon, Anne-Marie Moulin, Hugh McNaught, Guy Ouakil, Jean-Jacques Pocidalo, Kumar Suri Rajinder, Christopher Rutty, Professeur Sawadogo, Jill Scatoloni, William Sergeant, Thomas and Nancy Shaffer, Frank Shimada, Kamal Singhal, Philippe Stoeckel, François Vachon, Blaise Yanogo, Albert Zondgo, and Marcelin Zoungrana.

The Death
of a Disease

1

The Last

Victims

Burkina Faso, September 2000

Boureima Bagré is five years old. He lives with his family in the village of Seguedin, in the Nanoro district of this West African country. Burkina Faso means "land of honest people."

Boureima helps shepherd the family's donkeys and goats, but, unlike the other children, he does not tug or pull on the animals to coax them into their pen at the end of the day. He cannot play for long without sitting down. Mostly he leans against the adobe wall, watching his sisters, mother, and aunts as they gather around an enormous flat rock, each woman gripping a stone with both hands to pound millet for the evening meal. Boureima's left leg is withered and bent, and it turns out unnaturally from the knee. He limps when he walks.

Aïnata Kafando lives in the village of Sassa, in the district of Yako, in Burkina Faso. Aïnata, who is six, likes to stay next to her grandmother or near her father as he feeds millet into a machine that crushes it. The noise from the diesel motor that powers the machine, located halfway between their concession and the national highway, is deafening. Walking is not easy for Aïnata. Her foot is strapped into a metal caliper that holds her leg straight but hinders her movements.

Aïnata and Boureima are victims of polio, a fate that other Burkinabe children should be spared in the future. This little girl and boy are among the last reported cases of polio in the country. Aïnata was stricken by "the Crippler" in November 1997 and Boureima in August 1998.

From late 1997 to the summer of 1998, a polio epidemic swept the farmlands that extend from the suburbs of Ouagadougou to the districts of Nanoro and Yako, halfway between the capital city and the border with Mali. At the time this book was going to print, the last documented case of polio in Burkina Faso was that of Salam Kaboré, examined by a nurse from the Nanoro district on September 18, 1998.[1]

Burkina Faso, polio-free! For people who know this landlocked country, one of the poorest nations in the world, the news is hard to believe.

Statistics on the country's economy and health care speak for themselves: 81.5 percent of the population is illiterate. There is one doctor for every 25,000 inhabitants, and the gross national product is $240 per person. Burkina Faso is sixth from the bottom on the human development indicator. This index was established by the United Nations as a means of measuring human development; rankings are based on life expectancy, standard of living, and access to education. All these factors combined to make Burkina Faso especially fertile ground for the poliovirus to spread.

But the global eradication of polio is underway. The World Health Organization (WHO) has already certified the Americas, the Western Pacific Region, and Europe polio-free. From 1988 to 1999, the total number of cases worldwide fell dramatically: from an estimated 350,000 in 1988 to 7,141 reported in 1999; 2,979 in 2000; and 483 in 2001. The number of countries where polio is endemic has dropped steadily, from 50 in 1999 to 20 in 2000 and 7 in 2001.

Soon, the stories of all the Aïnatas, Boureimas, and Salams of this world will be history. Doctors in Burkina Faso, India, Peru, and Thailand will base their knowledge about polio on what they have gleaned from books—as is the case today for physicians in France, Canada, and the United States.

A disease as old as humanity is on the verge of being eliminated.

———

Boureima and Aïnata live in the Sahel.

Water is scarce here. Fetching water from the well is a task that falls to women and to girls as young as seven or eight. They carry jugs or pails balanced on their heads, sometimes walking hundreds of meters. When they arrive at the concession—a group of clay huts where a man lives with his wives, children, and members of his family—the women pour the water into large gourds.

Containers filled with water are placed on the ground, in the shadow of a wall. This is the water people use to wash their hands or cool their faces. This is the water they use for cooking and drinking. When no one is looking, sometimes the animals drink from the shallow containers to quench their thirst. Chickens—or "bicycle hens" as these skinny, long-legged fowl are known here—may wade across them.

It is likely that contaminated water in the gourds transmitted the poliovirus to Boureima and Aïnata. Or perhaps it was a pond, or contaminated food. The agent that causes polio is spread through contact with feces-contaminated water or food, or directly through saliva and the droplets exhaled by an infected person during the first two weeks following infection.

Once the poliovirus enters the body, it multiplies in the cells of the mucous membranes in the pharynx and intestines. The incubation period lasts from four to thirty-five days, but the first symptoms of the disease usually appear between seven and fourteen days after infection. The virus is excreted in the stool for three to six weeks. Polio is more stable than most viruses and can stay alive for several weeks in contaminated water or food. It is one of the most contagious viruses. When one member of a family is infected, nearly all the rest of the family becomes infected as well.

In concessions of the kind where Boureima and Aïnata live, outhouses and privies do not exist; the only alternative is the surrounding wilderness. The poliovirus excreted in the stools is transmitted by people, or carried on the hooves of animals that have come into contact with food or water for human consumption. It might enter the water of a pond where children fish, play, or drink. According to the WHO, one in five people across the planet lacks safe drinking water. Victims of polio are among this group.

Boureima and Aïnata were doubly unfortunate: first, because they were not exposed to the virus while nursing as babies. Breast milk usually contains antibodies that confer protection against polio. Antibodies are produced by the immune system when it is infected for the first time by a microbe. They remain in the immune system and defend the body against becoming infected again by the same microbe. A mother's antibodies pass through breast milk and protect her newborn baby for the first few weeks of life. If an infant is exposed to the poliovirus very early in life, his own immune system produces antibodies that will stay with him for the rest of his life, while the maternal antibodies protect him against this first infection.

Boureima and Aïnata were also unfortunate to be among the small minority of children who fell ill after infection by the poliovirus. In 90 percent of childhood cases, the virus causes no visible symptoms. Most of the time, the remaining 10 percent of children may experience headache, fever, a sore throat, or vomiting. The sore throat and vomiting are due to the proliferation of the virus in the upper digestive tract after it enters the mouth. Fever is the body's classic reaction to infection.

These symptoms are very common and, for children living in tropical climates, may have so many different causes that parents often seek traditional remedies or go to a healer. Usually they just wait for the symptoms to pass.

The Poliovirus

— The virion consists of a single strand of RNA containing genetic information and a protein coat.

— The poliovirus is a member of a larger family known as the Picornaviruses, which also includes rhinoviruses (influenza) and the hepatitis A virus.

— Polio belongs to the enterovirus subgroup, made up of over seventy viruses that infect the intestines.

— It is one of the smallest RNA viruses, measuring only 25–30 nm in diameter.

— Humans are its only natural host.

Depending on the type of virus, one child out of 100, 200, or 1,000 will be paralyzed. From the viewpoint of health authorities and the WHO, a single confirmed case of polio signals an epidemic, since for every declared case there are hundreds of healthy carriers of the virus.

The poliovirus moves silently from one child to the next over weeks and months before it cuts short the momentum of a young life. In developing countries, where hygiene is especially poor, patients are nearly always between two and five years old. The youngest children are protected by breastfeeding. Most people over age five have already been exposed to the virus.

Simandé Ouédraogo, the mother of Boureima, talks about the disease that struck down her son when he was three years old. She describes his first visit to the Health and Social Protection Center ("Centre de Santé et de Protection Sociale," CSPS) located in Seguedin, on August 21, 1998. The dispensary is a thirty-minute walk from the concession.

"I first knew Boureima was ill when he came down with a fever. I went to the health center and the health worker told me it was malaria. He gave my son a shot and told me to come back in the evening. When I came back, Boureima's fever was gone. They told me he was fine and gave me some tablets."

The nurse's assistant, a young man, made the following entry in Boureima's health record: "Temperature 38°C. Malaria without complications. Quinine injection." In tropical countries, the first symptoms of polio are often mistaken for malaria, the main cause of morbidity in regions such as Seguedin. To describe the signs of polio, local doctors speak of "malaria-like symptoms." In industrialized countries, they are referred to as "flu-like."

Misdiagnosing the onset of polio as malaria may have unfortunate consequences for patients. Often, people being treated for malaria are given an injection of quinine, which Boureima received. Intramuscular injections are an aggravating factor in the risk of polio-related paralysis. The best thing that can happen to a child like Boureima is to receive no treatment at all before paralysis is diagnosed, since treatment for an unexplained fever usually consists of injec-

tions of malaria drugs or antibiotics. Boureima's mother
continued:

"The fever had come back the next day. He had trouble
walking. He couldn't stand up. I went back to the health
center, where the nurse asked me if he had trouble walking

Never Again

Hello Doctor!

*I am sending you this child, who came to the CSPS
on 8/21/98 in my absence, with a fever of 38 °C. We of
course gave him a quinine injection.*

*This morning, the 22nd, his mother tells us he can-
not walk. After questioning, she told us this was well
before he came to the dispensary.*

We are sending him to you for an examination.

8/22/98
Signature

Letter of referral, excerpt from Boureima Bagré's health
record.

---

because of the shot. I told him no. He said I should go see
the doctor at the medical center in Nanoro."

On August 24, Simandé Ouédraogo, riding a bicycle with
Boureima on her back, made the twenty-two-kilometer journey on the dusty red dirt road that leads to the district medical center. The two doctors who work there are the only
physicians assigned to an area where 131,000 people live.
The district has fifteen CSPS run by nurses.

A doctor performed the Acute Flaccid Paralysis (AFP)
examination on Boureima. AFP is the primary symptom of
polio. With this form of paralysis, the muscles lose their
tone and strength and the limbs are "flaccid." The tendon

and skin reflexes disappear. By comparison, in so-called spastic paralysis, the limbs are stiff.

To perform this exam, the doctor had Boureima lie on his back and bend his legs with the knees touching. The left leg fell outward. The doctor bent and straightened the boy's legs, one at a time, to test the muscle tone, only to find that the boy's left leg had none. He brushed his finger along the arches of the boy's feet and his calves; there was no skin reflex from the left leg. Using a mallet, he tested the knee and ankle reflexes, which were very weak or entirely absent from the left leg. Finally, he grasped Boureima under the arms and lifted the boy, trying to make him walk, but Boureima's left leg bent to one side, his foot turned outward.

The doctor studied Boureima's health record. At the bottom of a page already filled with notes, he added three letters: AFP. He ruffled through the papers on his desk until he found a red pen, with which he noted the results of his examination:

> *AFP* (underlined three times)
> *Pain when standing. Bone-tendon reflexes absent from
>   both knees; no left arch reflex.*
> *No sign of diarrhea.*
> *Child never immunized.*
> *Massage and physical therapy at home.*
> *Take stool sample to be sent to the DMP* (Preventive
>   Medicine Division)

From a drawer in his desk, he extracted a form with the words *Acute Flaccid Paralysis Case Investigation Form* typed across the top. The World Health Organization distributes this form worldwide through each country's ministry of health. The child's AFP and other symptoms strongly suggested polio, but more evidence was needed to confirm the diagnosis. AFP may also be caused by enteroviruses other than the poliovirus, such as coxsackievirus or echovirus, and by bacteria, medicines, or even insect and reptile venom. Since polio was on the wane in Burkina Faso, more often than not cases of AFP were part of the clinical description of a neurological syndrome called Guillain-Barré syndrome, a disease thought to be caused by certain infections, an injection, or other causes, which generally disappears without any lasting ill-effects. The suspicion of Guillain-Barré syndrome explains the reaction of the nurse in Seguedin, who asked Boureima's mother if the child's paralysis appeared following a shot.

All cases of AFP are reported and investigated according to a detailed procedure defined by the WHO. A nurse will bring the form to the Preventive Medicine Division located in Ouagadougou, with two stool samples that must be kept refrigerated. The samples will be sent to a laboratory in Abidjan in the Ivory Coast, Burkina Faso's southwestern neighbor. This laboratory has been designated by the WHO as being able to detect the poliovirus and to identify the viral strain for several countries in West Africa. The results are sent to the country where the case was originally declared, which then reports cases of AFP and confirmed polio to the WHO.

Simandé Ouédraogo returned to the medical center on the afternoon of August 31. Boureima was kept under observation. He was in a coma. His fever rose to 40°C and his left side was paralyzed. He had bronchial pneumonia. The doctor wrote on his health record: "Referral to pediatrics ward, NHC" (National Hospital Center, Ouagadougou).

Says Boureima's mother: "The doctor did not tell me anything special. He just said I had to go to the hospital in Ouagadougou, so they could examine Boureima."

Simandé Ouédraogo never heard the doctor pronounce the word "polio." She does not know what germs are. When asked, she says she does not know what happened to her son. In her concession, surrounded by fields of maize, far removed from the city, no one knows how to read or write. The closest physical therapist is at least one hundred kilometers away. What could she do with the prescription for massages and physical therapy given by the doctor in Nanoro? This piece of paper was of no use.

The poliovirus was raging in Boureima's body. His immune system was not able to keep it from entering the bloodstream after it had multiplied in the cells of the mucous lining of his pharynx or intestines. The infectious agent entered his central nervous system and lodged in the cells where it grows best.

The poliovirus spreads to the gray matter formed by the nerve cells in the two anterior horns of the spinal cord and brain stem. This gray matter gives the disease its name: Poliomyelitis comes from the Greek word *polio*, meaning gray, *myelo*, meaning spinal cord, and *itis*, a suffix derived from Latin, which means "inflammation of" (as in meningitis, appendicitis, etc.). The virus spreads from the spinal

---

How the Virus Spreads in the Body

The poliovirus enters the body and spreads in one of two ways, or sometimes both:
— From the mucous of the pharynx, it reaches the tonsils and then the lymph nodes of the neck, and from here it enters the blood.
— From the mucous of the gastrointestinal tract, it reaches the lymph nodes of the small intestine and enters the bloodstream.

cord to the neurons that connect the spinal cord to the muscles; these are the "motor" neurons that enable us to move our arms, legs, diaphragm, and other muscles. Bundles of neurons make up the nerves that control a given muscle.

The poliovirus has a preference for the motor neurons; the virus multiplies there and damages the neurons. If all the neurons that make up a nerve controlling a certain muscle are destroyed, the muscle will be totally paralyzed. The muscle itself remains intact, but communication with the brain is cut off, and it no longer receives orders from the brain. If the virus destroys only one part of the neurons of a

---

Polio's Lasting Effects

Among children who suffer paralysis due to polio:

- 30 percent make a full recovery
- 30 percent are left with mild paralysis
- 30 percent have medium to severe paralysis
- 10 percent die

Source: L'interactif, Handicap International, June 1998.

---

nerve, the muscle will be weakened but still able to function.

The degree of paralysis depends on which neurons are affected and the amount of damage they sustain. In 79 percent of cases, the limbs are affected (spinal polio), most often the legs. The extensor muscles are damaged more often than are the flexors. If the virus reaches the medulla (bulbar polio), which controls the respiratory muscles and the diaphragm in particular, the disease can lead to death from asphyxiation. It may also cause the heart to fail. Bulbar polio represents 2 percent of cases. Bulbospinal polio, a combination of bulbar and spinal paralysis, accounts for 19 percent of cases.

The disease progresses differently in children and adults. The incubation period before the symptoms first appear is longer and fever is not as high for adults, but paralysis is more common and more severe. Mortality from polio is 2 to 5 percent among children, compared to 15 to 30 percent among adults.

There is no known treatment for polio. Nothing can stop the virus once it has invaded the body. Doctors can only wait, helping the patient as best they can until the immune system overpowers and eliminates the infectious agent.

Doctor Sawadogo is the head of the pediatrics ward at the Ouagadougou Hospital. He explains: "The children who come here with polio very often have other complications in addition to polio. They sometimes suffer from dehydration due to diarrhea or vomiting. In addition, they often present with neuromeningeal symptoms, or viral meningitis produced by the virus.

"We give them medicine to bring the fever down, prescribe bed rest, and start a multivitamin treatment with vitamins E and C. In children with polio, the course of the disease is unpredictable. Some recover nearly completely, while others suffer life-threatening breathing difficulties.

"Often, people will not tell us the truth about how long the child has been ill. They are afraid we will scold them for taking too long to bring him in. Many cases of paralysis are not reported, and we do not see the child until five or six years later."

After the disease has run its course, the victim's condition generally improves. Surviving intact neurons grow extensions that partially replace the damaged neurons. Certain muscles recover and function almost normally. Boureima recovered the full use of his right leg, which had been partially paralyzed with diminished reflexes when the doctor examined it. The paralysis in his left leg also became less severe.

Boureima's mother did not follow the Nanoro doctor's advice to bring Boureima to be examined by Doctor Sawadogo. She knew that this would involve taking a bus from Seguedin to Bouré on the national road and another vehicle from Bouré to Ouagadougou for a total cost, round-trip, of 3,000 CFA francs (about $4). She would need to locate the hospital, find a place to sleep and prepare meals, and pay the doctor's fee. The money, the difficulty, and the fear of the unknown added up to an insurmountable obstacle. Boureima had no further contact with the health center. At the marketplace, his mother found a small three-wheeled cart with a large handle. After a few months Boureima had learned to walk by leaning on the cart.

The results of the laboratory analyses of Boureima's stool sample are not filed in the records of the Preventive Medicine Division. His mother clearly remembers him giving the sample in Nanoro. The most likely explanation is that the cold chain was broken on the journey from the medical center in Nanoro to Abidjan. The samples were probably unusable and were at some point thrown away. Boureima's paralysis leaves no doubt as to whether he actually contracted polio, but since his case was not officially confirmed by a WHO-approved laboratory, he does not figure in the statistics.

With the addition of Boureima, the known number of cases of poliomyelitis in Burkina Faso in 1998, the last year in which the disease was reported, rises from four to five cases. Other children have probably been paralyzed or died of polio without ever seeing anyone at the CSPS or being reported by a nurse. Very often going to the dispensary involves walking for hours under the hot Sahel sun. The expense is another factor: the visit cost 200 CFA francs (the equivalent of 2 French francs, or around 30 cents) without counting the medicine. According to the Burkina Faso minister of health, the actual cost of a visit is ten times more, but 200 CFA francs is a significant sum for families who are almost completely self-subsistent and who sell very little of what their concession produces.

Aïnata's story differs from that of Boureima from a statistical point of view, since her type 1 poliovirus infection was officially confirmed in Abidjan. More important, Aïnata was fortunate to have a very special grandmother, Ruth Zongo. Aïnata's mother left the child with the family of her father, Jean Kafando, and she was put in the care of her grandmother, a woman of unusual determination, devotion, and perseverance. The family's standard of living was slightly higher than that of Boureima's family, as was proven by the fact that they owned a machine to grind millet. Aïnata lives just a few hundred meters from the road to Mali, not far from the city of Yako. Her family is less isolated than that of Boureima.

Ruth Zongo describes the first symptoms of Aïnata's illness, all of which are typical of polio. In November 1997, the little girl had fever and became "completely limp," according to her grandmother, who took her to the CSPS in Kalatanga. "The nurse scolded me, saying this was the type of situation that health-care workers did not want to see anymore. In the villages, they often organize immunization days to prevent many diseases, including the disease Aïnata got, which paralyzes the children's feet."

The grandmother is aware that "vaccines fight diseases" and "you need to vaccinate children when they are young, when their mothers still carry them on their backs," but Aïnata was not yet in her grandmother's care when she should have been vaccinated.

After the consultation at the CSPS, the grandmother

traveled with Aïnata to Nanoro, where she waited one week for a stool sample to be taken. After waiting four days, she was told that the little girl's illness was serious, and she was given a referral to the pediatrics ward at the Ouaga-dougou Hospital.

The patient registry of Dr. Sawadogo's ward mentions Aïnata's arrival on December 16, 1997. The staff performed the usual examinations and sent the child and her grandmother to the physical rehabilitation center in Ouagadougou.

The grandmother says: "They explained to us where we should go. We made many detours, but finally I found the place where they care for children with handicaps. We stayed there for a month and a half."

Aïnata began physical therapy. Her grandmother recalls that during the sessions, a physical therapist applied ban-dages and had the little girl use an apparatus that would teach her to walk while holding her leg straight.

"The health-care worker who cared for Aïnata told me he had been called away to an athletic competition for one month and that he would not be able to take care of her anymore. He told me we could not wait for him to come back and sent us to Koudougou to continue the therapy."

Ruth Zongo had taken Aïnata to Nanoro, some 30 kilo-meters west of Sassa, their village. Ruth had taken her to Ouagadougou, 110 kilometers to the southeast. Now she set off for a new destination, 97 kilometers to the west of the capital city.

"While she was at the rehabilitation center in Koudou-gou, Aïnata received massages," says Ruth. "She had to ride a bike with her feet strapped onto the pedals. She also learned how to walk with crutches. We stayed there three and a half months."

The grandmother and granddaughter had been away from their village five months. For all this time, they had to find a place to sleep, food to eat, and money to pay for Aïnata's care. A special fitted caliper with a knee piece was custom-made for Aïnata's right leg. The device and two crutches cost 12,000 CFA francs (about $16), a sacrifice for Aïnata's family.

Aïnata is one of an estimated ten to twenty million people in the world who live with the aftereffects of polio.

2

A Lifetime

Burden

Burkina Faso, September 2000

More than two years have gone by since the summer 1998 polio epidemic in Burkina Faso. Aïnata has grown. Her grandmother, tired and unwell, was not able to take her to the rehabilitation center to have her caliper adjusted. The shoe on the caliper is now too small for a foot that has grown. The knee piece is inches below the little girl's knee, and she can no longer bend her leg.

Ruth Zongo's efforts were not in vain, however. They have changed Aïnata's prospects for the future. The little girl limps, but she walks upright. She has learned how to compensate for her paralysis by using other muscles. Her leg is not deformed or atrophied and she does not suffer from sclerosis in her joints. If she is able to have new calipers fitted as she grows, which is likely, she will be able to live a very nearly normal life.

Of the six last known polio victims in Burkina Faso, Aïnata is probably the only one fortunate enough to have received physical therapy and a caliper.

Boureima's mother did not take him to Ouagadougou.

A third child by the name of Adama Ouédraogo first

came to the Saint Camille Medical Center, on the outskirts of Ouagadougou, on May 18, 1998. After treating the boy, the medical staff referred him to a rehabilitation center located on the same grounds. Adama was given a few sessions of physical therapy by an orthopedic specialist, but his parents decided to return to their village, Manga, putting their trust in traditional medicine.

A fourth child, Boubacar Ouédraogo, from the suburbs of Ouagadougou, was examined by Dr. Sawadogo on June 14. Dr. Sawadogo referred him to the Burkina National Center for Orthopedic Devices. On September 10, the Center's head physician diagnosed the boy with deformities of the knee and outward rotation of the right foot. He prescribed a caliper. A physical therapist took the measurements to have a device fitted for Boubacar's leg. The family was asked to pay in advance for the device, and did not. The device was never made and the child never returned to the center.

A fifth child, Saïdou Gadiaga, came with his mother to the Paul 6 Medical Center in the suburbs of Ouagadougou on July 23. He was scheduled for a medical visit the next day, but did not come. A nun who was also a nurse tried to find the boy and discovered that he and his mother had set out that day for their village, located north of the capital city. Saïdou died on the journey home.

The sixth and last child of the group, Salam Kaboré, was examined at the Nanoro Medical Center on September 18, after which there is no record of the boy.

Aïnata began physical therapy at the Burkina National Center for Orthopedic Devices in Ouagadougou. Dr. Blaise Yanogo, head physician at the center, explains the paralytic sequelae of polio: "With polio, certain muscles in the limb become flaccid, or limp. For example, if the muscles that pull the toes downward are working, but those that pull it upward are not, the foot will tend to drop toward the ground. When this happens, polio victims cannot walk properly because they cannot put their heel on the ground. If the situation is left untreated, the tendons at the back of the foot retract and the foot cannot resume a normal position. This is referred to as an equinus foot and is typical of polio. The same type of deformity may occur in the arm."

In the least severe cases of paralysis of one leg, the affected limb becomes atrophied through lack of activity, while the other limb continues to grow normally. One leg is shorter than the other and the person limps, leaning to one side, which leads to deformities of the spine.

In the most serious cases, when both legs are affected, polio victims put their weight on their knees and move about using their hands and arms. The limbs become atrophied below the knee and the joints are in angular positions.

In developing countries such as Burkina Faso, life for people with disabilities is often very difficult. In Nanoro, a group of young adults who have severe sequelae from polio founded an association to attempt to find the means to live a normal life. It's called the Relwandé Association of the Disabled of Nanoro. Alfred Saté Conduma, president of the association, explains:

"We created an association of polio victims in order to ask for help. We suffer greatly. Some of us have to drag ourselves along the ground on all fours. We have no wheelchairs for people with paralysis; we don't even have crutches. We've asked everywhere for help to create a center where we could work as a community and earn enough to live on, without needing to beg for food."

But begging is what the future holds for many victims of polio in developing countries. Countless martyrs to the disease dot the sidewalks and roadways of Dakar, Nairobi,

New Delhi, and Saigon. The luckiest victims have a wheel-chair, while others drag their deformed and atrophied legs behind them.

Very often, the lasting paralysis caused by polio is a source of shame. Albert Zondgo is a physical therapist at the Rehabilitation and Orthopedics Center of Kaya, located one hundred kilometers northeast of Ouagadougou. "Often," he says, "people don't want anyone to see their handicapped children, so they keep them hidden. The children don't go to school, can't get married, and have no other choice but to beg. It was only recently that parents began to realize that we can do something to help children who have had polio.

"When the father is educated (because it's the father who decides) he knows that polio is a disease like any other, and that we can treat it. But when he lives in the brush and does not understand illnesses and medicine, he thinks somebody put a curse on him. Even today, we have to explain to some parents that their child has not been cursed, and that we can give the child physical therapy. Unfortunately, the families often wait too long before they come to see us, either because they don't know about the center, or because they have no money."

The center in Kaya receives funding from Marija, a Swiss nongovernmental organization. The buildings and grounds are spacious and well kept. The center has various kinds of equipment for physical therapy, all in good condition. Patients can stay in the rooms at the center for several weeks. Except for a few patients who come from relatively prosperous families who own a business or shop, the patients at the Kaya Center pay only a portion of the actual cost of care. Aïnata did not enjoy such fine conditions in the public rehabilitation centers of Ouagadougou and Koudougou, which are run by the Burkina Faso Ministry of Health.

When a polio victim comes to the center a long time

after being ill with polio, the staff must first correct the deformities left by the disease. "Monday is the day we make plaster casts," says Albert Zondgo. "We apply a cast and leave it in place for a week or two, depending on the situation: two weeks for severe retraction; otherwise it's one week. Once the cast is removed, we use a wooden wedge to move the limb slightly, and then we make another plaster cast. When we do this over and over, the position of the limb gradually changes. The treatment may take one to two months. The patients are hospitalized at the center during this time."

The physical therapist explains that he has to complete the repositioning of the knee of a twenty-year-old student, Zouanda Alémata, before classes start again, because she must return to school. Another patient, Diallo Salamata, has been at the center for almost two months. His equinus foot has disappeared and the arch of his foot is once again perpendicular to his leg.

Once patients' retractions and deformities have been corrected, they can begin physical therapy. Regardless of a patient's age, the goal is the same. "When a child has had polio," says Albert Zondgo, "certain muscles are generally preserved and can make up for those that don't work. We must teach the child to use these muscles to compensate for the others, and they will be strengthened."

Rehabilitation is intended to accomplish this. Braces, or calipers, help the weakened leg to support the weight of the body, guide the bending of joints, and correct poor positioning, preventing the development of deformities. In just six months without the caliper or brace, retractions may appear or reappear.

For the most serious deformities, surgery is the only way a polio victim may walk again. During the operation, which takes place under general anesthesia, the surgeon stretches the retracted tendons by cutting away approximately two-thirds of their thickness so that the remaining one-third will then stretch. This technique can be used, for example, to quickly correct an equinus foot. The surgeon can also operate on bones and joints, for example, to reduce and stabilize a dislocation of the hip. Such complex operations, however, are for specialists only and require sophisticated surgical facilities.

The doctors in Nanoro and at the hospital in Ouagadougou do not mention the possibility of surgery for polio victims; neither do the physical therapists in the rehabilitation centers of Ouagadougou and Kaya. Surgery is not a realistic option for most polio victims in the world because it is beyond their means.

The physical suffering caused by polio is not always limited to the immediate aftereffects of the disease. Adults who had polio when they were children may see their sequelae worsen and their paralysis spread decades after their condition has stabilized and they have completed rehabilitation or undergone surgery.

Marie Héraud, a French patient, describes what happened to her:

"I was born in December 1925 and contracted polio when I was eight months old. My right leg was severely affected, but until I was forty-seven, I could walk ten kilometers; I could stroll through a museum all afternoon. Suddenly I had trouble walking down stairs, then trouble walking. When I was fifty-four, I started using a cane and by the time I was sixty, I needed two of them. This is how I walked for ten years. Then I couldn't hold myself up on canes anymore and switched to a walker with wheels and finally to a motorized wheelchair.

"Today I can walk one hundred meters with a walker. I can stand up for one minute. I have to lie down fifteen hours a day due to fatigue."[1]

Post-polio syndrome affects 25 to 40 percent of polio victims and appears some twenty-five to forty years after the onset of acute polio. It is not entirely clear what causes the syndrome. Today, specialists have ruled out the hypothesis of a sudden reawakening of virus that may not have been eliminated by the immune system, remaining dormant for dozens of years. The most likely explanation is the one put forward in 1981 by David Wiechers and Susan Hubbell: the nerve extensions that enabled the nerves to become partly functional after the acute phase of the disease are not as strong as the original motor neurons. They become tired, wear out, and disappear over time. Various treatments for post-polio syndrome are being experimented with, but so far the results have not been conclusive.

The March of Dimes, the private charity that played a decisive role in the battle against polio in the United States in the 1940s and 1950s, estimates that today there are 250,000 polio victims with post-polio syndrome in the United States; 40,000 in Germany; 30,000 in Japan; 24,000 in France; and 12,000 in Canada and the United Kingdom, and that the number of victims worldwide will reach four to eight million.

Even if the goal of the Global Polio Eradication Initiative—launched by the WHO in 1988—is met and the poliovirus is eliminated from the planet in the twenty-first century, the burden of this disease will continue to grow for decades.

3

A Virus

with a Long

History

Egypt, 2000 B.C. and Europe, Twentieth Century

Roma the Guardian was a priest of the Egyptian goddess Astarte. He is one of the central figures on a stele on display at the Glyptothek Museum in Copenhagen, a stone slab dating back to the eighteenth pharaonic dynasty (sixteenth to thirteenth centuries B.C.). He leans on a staff, his right leg withered and dangling, his foot in the *equinus* position. Roma is the oldest documented victim of poliomyelitis.

In his book *A History of Poliomyelitis,* John Paul of Yale University, who was a polio researcher and one of the foremost authorities on the history of the disease, discusses what may have been cases of paralytic poliomyelitis in the works of Hippocrates. John Paul believes that the disease was endemic during classical Greco-Roman times.[1] Although other researchers' conclusions may vary, they all agree on one essential point: the poliovirus is at least three thousand years old.

Closer to our time, polio has left traces in art of the sixteenth-century Flemish school. Two crippled figures appear in one of Pieter Bruegel the Elder's paintings, *The Fight between Carnival and Lent* (1559). One figure, who has a maimed leg, walks with a wooden crutch. The other moves forward on his hands, his shrunken and bent legs strapped to splints and dragging behind him. Although this artistic testimony is not formal proof of poliomyelitis, it strongly suggests that both suffered from the disease.

Polio went almost unnoticed during the centuries when famine, the plague, smallpox, and other diseases wiped out entire sectors of the population. In 1789, Michael Underwood, an English physician, was the first to describe "debility of the lower extremities," which he attributed to "teething" or "fever." The illness appeared to be rare and was not considered a serious problem.

At about this time, polio struck a small boy, later to become its first famous victim. Sir Walter Scott (1771–1832), born in Edinburgh, lost the use of one of his legs when he was very young. His parents decided to send him to stay with his grandparents in the Highlands. To keep the handicapped child's mind occupied, his aunt and grandmother sang him ballads and told him tales and ancient legends. As he grew up, Scott, imbued with nostalgia for the past, revealed a talent for writing. Among his many works is the immensely popular novel, *Ivanhoe*.

In 1840, Jacob von Heine, a German physician, noted a significant number of cases of "infantile paralysis" and described the clinical symptoms. Thirty years later, in 1870, Alfred Vulpian, a French neurologist, concluded that the disease was contagious and wrote a description that is still valid today: "This atrophic paralysis is apparently an acute infectious disease, which results from an infection of the body that is usually localized in a limited region of the spinal cord."

In 1881, a polio epidemic broke out in a small town in northern Sweden. Some twenty children suddenly came down with diarrhea, malaise, and fever. Six years later, in Stockholm, forty-four children were stricken with a similar illness. Three of them died. Their doctor, the pediatrician Oskar Medin, carried out autopsies on the bodies and found that the disease had attacked the nerves of the spinal cord and the base of the brain. His observation of these two series of cases led him to conclude that the disease was infectious.

In 1888, S. Cordier, a French physician, retrospectively described thirteen cases of infantile atrophic paralysis that occurred in the summer of 1885 in the village of Sainte-Foy l'Argentière, near the city of Lyon. Five of the children were less than seven months old when they fell ill.

Poliomyelitis had always been endemic, with sporadic cases observed in children. Now, at the close of the nineteenth century, polio was causing epidemics. Outbreaks paralyzed hundreds of people. The fear of polio spread.

In 1894, the disease caused an outbreak in Vermont when 119 children were diagnosed with polio. Another epidemic in Sweden in 1905 killed hundreds of children and left nearly one thousand paralyzed. A Swedish physician, Ivar Wickman, put forward the hypothesis that this was a contagious disease; individuals carrying the infectious agent transmitted it to others.

A more intense scientific study of poliomyelitis began in 1909, when the Austrian physician, Karl Landsteiner, and his colleagues, Erwin Popper and Constantin Levaditi, successfully reproduced the disease in their laboratory by taking a spinal cord sample from a child who had died of polio and injecting it into a baboon and a rhesus monkey. A few days later, the baboon was found dead, while the hind legs of the rhesus monkey were paralyzed. The biologists filtered the injected liquid and found that the agent of infection was not a bacterium, which would not have passed through the filter, but a much smaller microbe.

The First Vaccines

In China, as early as the Renaissance, doctors sometimes blew pulverized scabs of smallpox sores into people's noses to protect them from contracting the disease.

In 1796, the English physician Edward Jenner noticed that milkmaids who milked cows with cowpox, caused by the vaccinia virus, were protected against smallpox. This gave him the idea of inoculating individuals with extracts from the pustules of cows.

Louis Pasteur became famous when, in 1885, he injected young Joseph Meister with a rabies virus that had been attenuated in his laboratory. He thus invented the first modern vaccine and coined the term vaccine in honor of the vaccinia virus used by Jenner.

Soon after this, the scientists injected extracts of the dead baboon's nerve tissue into the surviving rhesus monkey. The animal had become resistant to the disease, no matter what dose was injected. It had acquired immunity to poliomyelitis. If an initial infection provided protection against reinfection, the scientists reasoned, it should be possible to develop a vaccine. They decided they would need to administer attenuated or killed viruses to elicit an immune response, a method that was already used to prevent smallpox and rabies.

However, no one yet understood how poliomyelitis was transmitted. The scientific community wondered whether flies or cockroaches transported the virus. Until the late 1930s, the general opinion was that it penetrated the body through the nose, because in the early stages of the disease the virus can be detected in the throat. Some physicians suggested sectioning the olfactory nerves to prevent its spreading to the brain and the spinal cord. Experimental nasal sprays caused some children to lose their sense of smell forever, but did not give them protection from polio.

In 1916, a devastating polio epidemic sent waves of panic throughout the northeastern United States. Some 27,000 people were paralyzed and 6,000 died.

During the centuries prior to these epidemics, the poliovirus was endemic, infecting nearly all children in the few months after they were born, when they were still protected by the antibodies received through their mothers' milk. Some children who had not undergone this natural immunization process contracted the disease with varying degrees of severity. The symptoms of polio went unnoticed in the midst of the transitory fevers and gastroenteritis that often affect young children. The epidemics wrought havoc as they broke out among the most protected social classes of the industrialized countries. The disease also struck adolescents and adults, often in a more severe form than that affecting young children.

The United States and the Scandinavian countries, known to have high standards of hygiene, were those most seriously hit by polio. The public was alarmed to discover that not only did good hygiene fail to prevent this infectious disease, it even appeared to spread it further. Efforts such as sterilizing tap water and boiling milk for children seemed futile; it was almost as if polio epidemics were a perverse side effect of cleanliness.

In French-speaking countries, polio became known as "la maladie de la savonnette" (the cake of soap disease). A specialist at the Pasteur Institute is rumored to have said, "If all children wiped their slices of bread and butter against the wall before they ate them, polio would be less frequent."

4

The People

versus Polio

United States, Mid-Twentieth Century

Polio was not the most deadly nor the most contagious disease, but it was easily the most dreaded disease in North America in the first half of the twentieth century.

Polio outbreaks amounted to scattered pockets of disease in the United States until the epidemic of 1916 in the northeastern part of the country marked a horrifying peak, with 2,448 deaths in New York City alone by October.

The Department of Health ordered quarantines for polio victims and their families; windows had to be screened, bed linen disinfected, and household pets banned from a patient's room. Children under age sixteen were not allowed to travel from July 18 to October 3 unless they had a certificate stating that their homes were polio-free.[1] City authorities imposed the same precautions that had been effective in limiting diseases such as the plague or influenza.

At the same time, shiploads of immigrants were arriving at Ellis Island and many public health experts and New Yorkers, in the grip of fear, looked about, anxious to lay blame and identify the source of this mysterious illness. City health officials were convinced that polio was associated with poor hygiene and crowded urban living conditions and blamed the spread of polio mainly on immigrants. Equating disease with poverty and dirt, they responded to the threat of polio by emphasizing cleanliness, control of insects, and quarantines, targeting immigrant ghettos, slums, and tenements, and imposing drastic restrictions.

These measures were, however, ineffective. Polio was a predominantly middle-class disease, mostly affecting developed countries and, in particular, communities with the highest standards of hygiene.

After the terrible epidemic of 1916, not a year went by without an epidemic somewhere in the United States. The post–World War II years were especially frightening, with an unprecedented and inexplicable rise in the number of cases and in the severity of the disease. In 1940, over 10,000 cases were reported; in 1946, the number of cases grew to 25,000. The worst epidemic in the history of the United States occurred during the summer of 1952, with nearly 60,000 polio cases and 3,000 deaths reported.

By comparison, at the end of 1957, following the widespread introduction of the Jonas Salk vaccine, only 5,000 cases were reported and the number dropped to 3,000 by 1960.

The country's northern neighbor was hit even harder on a per capita basis. Canada experienced its most severe epidemic wave from 1946 to 1953, peaking with a national polio crisis in 1953. Manitoba faced what local papers referred to as the "world's worst" polio epidemic, with a record 244 cases per week in August 1953. According to Canadian historian and polio specialist Christopher Rutty,[2] for the 1952 epidemic, the U.S. case notification rate was 36.2 per 100,000, compared to a national case rate of 60 per 100,000 in Canada during the 1953 epidemic. The 1953 epidemic brought polio to the fore as a major public health problem in Canada.

Numbers, however, do little to convey the terrible fear that swept North America. No one had any idea where this unpredictable infection came from. Epidemiologists were at a loss to explain how it was transmitted. There seemed to be neither rhyme nor reason to the randomness with which it suddenly struck and paralyzed, most often children. Every summer, with the advent of "polio season," fearful parents forbade children from going to the swimming pool, the fairground, or the movie theater; camping trips were canceled and parents were warned to keep their children bathed, rested, and away from crowds. The everyday pleasures of summertime were suddenly off-limits, and everyone lived in fear of indulging in some illicit pleasure that might make them come down with polio, "a ritual taboo against sensual indulgence in times of crisis," as Jane Smith put it in *Patenting the Sun: Polio and the Salk Vaccine*.[3]

In 1921 polio struck its most famous victim, Franklin Delano Roosevelt, who fell ill while vacationing on Campobello Island off the coast of Maine. He was thirty-nine years old. It took two weeks and three doctors to diagnose the disease, even though the 1916 epidemic was still fresh in the public mind. The Roosevelt family did not fit people's idea of who might get polio.

Even more than the devastation of the disease, the story of Franklin Roosevelt holds the key to understanding the overwhelming popular reaction to polio in America, the mobilization of individuals who channeled their energies into raising money to care for polio victims, support research, make it possible to develop a vaccine, and rein in a terrifying epidemic.

Franklin Roosevelt changed the image of polio, which could no longer be characterized as a dirty disease afflicting poor immigrants and children, and polio transformed

Franklin Roosevelt, both personally and politically. As a polio survivor and living proof of triumph in the face of adversity, a fundamental American value, Roosevelt was both heroic and approachable in the eyes of common citizens. When Eleanor Roosevelt was asked whether her husband's illness had affected his mentality, she replied: "The answer is 'Yes.' Anyone who has gone through great suffering is bound to have a greater sympathy and understanding of the problems of mankind."[4]

Roosevelt, often referred to affectionately as FDR, sought to be a champion for polio victims without appearing to be a victim of the disease. He believed that if voters saw him as handicapped, they would think of him as weak. Although he was permanently paralyzed from the hips down, he was almost never photographed in his wheelchair or in a way that made it appear he could not stand or walk. It is a miracle of American political journalism that the White House press corps cooperated in this deception. A touching reminder of this, and of slow changes in public attitudes toward the handicapped, is the new statue of FDR in his wheelchair, which was recently installed in Washington, D.C.

The physical handicap that could have disqualified Roosevelt from politics transformed him and gave him a special qualification for leadership.[5] He managed to turn his liability into an asset. In 1928, just seven years after he was stricken by polio, he ran for governor of New York and won, going on to serve two terms. He was elected to the presidency of the United States an unprecedented four times and is widely regarded as one of the most skillful and popular American politicians of the twentieth century. For many people, Roosevelt's name is synonymous with the New Deal, a program he engineered as soon as he took office (during the famous One Hundred Days) to pull the country out of the Great Depression that followed the stock market crash of 1929. He is also remembered alongside Winston Churchill, representing the Allied powers in the Second World War.

Roosevelt's presidency (1932–1945) gave a tremendous boost to the fight against polio. In 1938, he prompted the creation of the National Foundation for Infantile Paralysis (NFIP), with the mission of finding a cure for polio. Roosevelt's longtime friend and law partner Basil O'Connor was made its president. O'Connor was to lead the NFIP for the rest of his life and was unquestionably the "producer" who made it work, always seeing to it that the foundation's machinery was well oiled and in working order, regardless of the scale of its operations.

The NFIP's goals were to support research, professional education, patient care, and polio prevention. The foundation wanted to ensure that no polio patient would be denied the best available treatment due to lack of funds. In addition, it intended to keep the public well informed about the disease and how to deal with it. In the early 1950s this foundation, run entirely on private contributions, spent ten times more on polio research than the U.S. National Institutes of Health.

In its heyday, roughly from 1941 to 1955, the organization was perceived by many as a public institution, and yet it was fueled by the contributions of the "middle of the middle class" and volunteers who were not likely to be solicited by the more high-brow Junior League. The NFIP was a grass-roots organization, with a unique and phenomenally successful structure. Three thousand NFIP local chapters were staffed by some 90,000 volunteers, who were supervised by five paid regional directors. An additional two million volunteers worked to collect money during the annual fund drive held each January. All NFIP operations were overseen by the national headquarters in New York, in the same office building at 120 Broadway where Basil O'Connor had his law office.

Prior to the establishment of the NFIP in 1938 and its phenomenal fund-raising drives, Basil O'Connor and the Warm Springs Foundation had begun organizing charity balls to celebrate the president's birthday, which was January 30. The Birthday Balls were intended to help finance a center for polio victims in Warm Springs, Georgia, a spot dear to Franklin Roosevelt's heart. Warm Springs was FDR's largest investment, one of over $200,000, and consumed more than one-third of his personal fortune. The balls began in 1934, when Roosevelt's popularity was at its peak. Postmasters (being appointed postmaster was a political plum) in each community were named honorary chairmen of the local Birthday Ball Committee; they were to raise money and ensure attendance at the ball.[6]

In the first year, six thousand balls were organized, bringing in over one million dollars. From 1934 to 1937, the ball's slogan was "To dance so that others may walk." During this same period of time, the balls raised a total of $3,362,000. Local committees kept 70 percent of the proceeds and spent these sums to help victims of polio.

In January 1938, the newly created NFIP procured the help of radio announcer and vaudeville star Eddie Cantor to launch its first fund-raising drive. Cantor urged listeners to contribute to the fight against polio and asked them to send a dime directly to the president. As the coins poured in, he dubbed the campaign "the March of Dimes," a play on the title of a popular newsreel at the time called "the March of Time."

Workers in the White House mailroom, which had to hire fifty extra postal clerks to handle the avalanche of mail in response to Cantor's appeal, complained that the U.S. government had nearly stopped functioning because they

---

What Could You Buy with a Dime?

In 1938, in small-town America, a dime would buy two ice-cream cones, two twelve-ounce bottles of Royal Crown Cola, two full-size candy bars, half a gallon of gasoline, a child's admission to the movies, two copies of the daily paper, or a good cigar. A haircut at the barber shop cost forty-five cents. If your mother gave you fifty cents, that left a nickel—or half a dime—for a draft root beer at the local drugstore soda fountain.

---

could not find the official White House mail among all those dimes.

The new foundation raised $1.8 million in 1938, of which $268,000 arrived in the White House mail one dime at a time: millions of dimes! Each year the sums raised by the foundation grew steadily, and, in spite of the war, in 1945 amounted to nearly $20 million.

After Eddie Cantor's broadcast, radio and film stars were eager to join the cause. The place of collection moved from the overburdened White House mailroom to movie theaters; Hollywood celebrities made short films, to be shown in the theater before the main feature, in which they urged people to reach into their pockets and fish out a dime.

In addition to the outpouring of dimes, the NFIP's permanent staff of publicity experts devised myriad ways of raising money. Their gimmicks made use of radio (and, later, television), poster children, and Mothers' March volunteers, housewives who carried cans with slots in them for the dimes, going house-to-house in their neighborhoods.

Specific appeals were designed for different target groups—adolescents, parents, grandparents, and so forth. Schoolchildren were asked to collect dimes and were rewarded by having their names put on a special honor roll if all the slots on their collection cards were filled; grandparents were told to send their grandchildren out of the room and then asked to think about what a terrible loss it would be if anything happened to them. In 1943, Mary Pickford, star of the silent screen, was appointed honorary director of NFIP women volunteers. From that time on, women became the March of Dimes' main resource, in part because they had to take up the baton while American men were off fighting in the war in Europe.

The March of Dimes was extraordinarily successful at raising huge amounts of money. Between 1938 and 1959, it raised a total of $622 million and spent half this to pay for the care of polio patients—medical, hospital, and rehabilitation expenses. It also spent $55 million on polio-related research and $33 million on polio education services for health care professionals, including nurses and physical therapists. In 1954, the year of the field trial to test Jonas Salk's vaccine, involving close to two million children, the foundation received nearly $68 million in donations.

The NFIP's fund-raising campaigns consistently dwarfed the efforts of most other voluntary health organizations; only the American Red Cross raised more dollars, and its success was part of the war effort. The campaigns, however, caused some polio researchers whose work it financed to feel ill-at-ease because of the NFIP's fund-raising and publicity methods.

The foundation solicited the help of celebrities, from Jack Benny to Judy Garland to Helen Hayes, whose daughter had died of polio. It also used scare tactics such as a terrifying film called *The Crippler*, in which polio is personified as a cackling, sinister figure lurking around playgrounds, ready to prey on children. Any means were justified to convince people to reach into their pocketbooks. Polio researcher John Paul compares the creation of the NFIP to "the sudden appearance of a fairy godmother of quite mammoth proportions who thrived on publicity." He explains how the polio cause became a crusade through the publicity efforts by the NFIP; polio research, he writes, became "a holy quest."

In addition to raising money, the NFIP also won the loyalty of all those who made contributions to it—whether great or small. Their actions meant that they were buying into a mutual assistance policy of sorts; if one day polio hit their families, they would have somewhere to turn. Whenever a scientific advancement was reported in the press or a community obtained an iron lung, the newspaper articles underlined that "this was made possible by *your* contribution."

The NFIP wanted to be sure anyone with polio who needed help could get it. Roughly half the donations it received went to the local community where the money was raised, to provide for the hospitalization and care of patients with polio; the rest was spent on professional training, assistance during epidemics, and to fund research for better treatment and a vaccine. In the postwar years, as the rise in the number of polio cases dovetailed with the baby boom, many new parents were eager to contribute to the cause. Parenthood suddenly made them directly concerned.

With the widespread use of the polio vaccines, the National Foundation (now known as the March of Dimes, having adopted the name of its annual campaign) was essentially out of a job. In the 1960s it shifted its focus to combating birth defects.

The fear of polio, compassion for the victims, and people's hope of finding a vaccine had driven this great popular movement. Polio was a national cause and money was raised by massive public mobilization, but the National

Foundation for Infantile Paralysis was an entirely private charity (albeit promoted by the president).

As the foundation itself points out, it is the only national health organization to have succeeded in helping defeat the disease it set out to conquer.

5

Freed

from the

Iron Lung

Europe, 1952–1954

In 1952, a polio epidemic in Denmark gave rise to an invention that changed the lives of polio victims suffering from respiratory complications and revolutionized emergency room techniques throughout the world.

Beginning in the mid-1930s, patients in danger of respiratory paralysis were placed in iron lungs, enormous metal boxes that enclosed the entire body up to the neck. Inside, the alternation between sub-atmospheric and atmospheric pressure caused the thoracic cage to move and kept the patient breathing. The machine was first developed by Dr. Philip Drinker and his team at the Harvard School of Public Health to provide assistance to premature babies and newborns in respiratory distress. It was improved and developed by the Warren Collins Corporation in the United States, which produced the machine commercially for polio victims. Officially known as the Drinker Respirator, it was soon

referred to as the iron lung, a name that helped conjure up
the terror that polio inspired in the public's mind.

During the 1952 polio epidemic, hospital physicians in
Copenhagen could scarcely cope with the number of patients
with respiratory paralysis. Only a few iron lungs were available, and these were insufficient in both number and efficacy to prevent death by asphyxiation.

A Danish physician, Dr. Henry Lassen, and his colleague,
Dr. Bjorn Ibsen, an anesthetist, suggested treating these patients by using a technique that had been employed with
success in surgery. A rubber tube was inserted through the
patient's mouth to the trachea to allow air to enter the lungs.
Someone at the patient's bedside applied manual pressure
to a balloon containing a mixture of air with oxygen so that
the air entered and left the lungs according to a natural pat-
tern of inhaling and exhaling.

The main drawback with this technique was that patients required assistance for days and even weeks. The advantage was that the patient's respiratory passageway could
be cleared of secretions through the tube, thereby preventing asphyxiation. Medical staff worked day and night to help
patients breathe. Students took turns pedaling bicycles
whose chains worked the machines.

Soon it became clear, however, that the tube to the lungs
could not be left in the patient's mouth for more than a few
days. The doctors then suggested performing a tracheotomy,
a surgical incision in the trachea through which is inserted
a cuffed tube that is hooked up to a mechanical respirator.
A tracheotomy establishes direct access to the bronchi, and
the tube can be left in place for a long period of time. It is
more comfortable for patients and prevents the airways from
being clogged up with secretions. Doctors used penicillin,
the first antibiotic, which had recently become available,

to prevent the risk of infection through the opening of the airways.

Doctors and engineers combined their efforts to improve on these "home-made" devices and develop more sophisticated artificial respirators on an industrial scale. One of these new machines was the Engström Respirator, the "Rolls Royce of artificial respiration" according to Dr. Jean-Jacques Pocidalo, who helped introduce the respirator in France. "It was met with much-deserved success in Europe," he said.

In the mid-1950s, the French health authorities, aware of the ravages wrought by polio epidemics in the Scandinavian countries, braced themselves, expecting the worst. Dr. Pierre Lépine, a polio specialist at the Pasteur Institute, asked Dr. Pierre Mollaret, who held the chair of Infectious Diseases at the Claude Bernard Hospital in Paris, to take steps to prepare to care for the most seriously affected patients.

Physicians in Paris knew about the Engström Respirators but no one had experience with using them for long periods of time. Pierre Mollaret, together with Jean-Jacques Pocidalo and others, spent the winter of 1953–1954 drawing up plans for a medical center equipped to care for a large number of polio victims suffering from respiratory paralysis. Ultramodern wards were equipped with brand-new Engström Respirators imported from Denmark and Sweden. An oxygen distribution unit was set up in the basement of the center.

To regulate the ventilation provided by the respirators, biologists developed a way to rapidly dose the amounts of oxygen and carbon dioxide in the patients' blood. The doctors prepared to perform tracheotomies. Nurses and doctors practiced using the respirators on dogs that had been anesthetized and paralyzed with curare. Their endeavors were rewarded. It was possible, for the first time, to provide patients suffering from respiratory distress with continuous mechanical ventilation. The iron lungs were stored in the back rooms of the care center.

When the expected epidemic hit France in September 1954, the well-trained teams were ready to receive patients for treatment at the center, now known as the Pasteur-Lassen Center. Their preparations had not been in vain. There were 2,000 polio victims in France in 1954, but mortality rates were not as high as those in northern Europe.

"Being able to anticipate events such as these means we can change the evolution of techniques, even in medicine," said Jean-Jacques Pocidalo.

The experience acquired by the staff at the Pasteur-Lassen Center spread throughout France. Other large hospitals were able to use the new practice of continuous artificial respiration, known as respiratory resuscitation, for all cases of respiratory distress. These changes were eventually introduced in major hospitals worldwide.

Respiratory resuscitation, a technique developed to treat polio, has become a routine practice to which generations of patients and accident victims owe their lives. The path taken by all who have joined in the fight against polio is dotted with such landmark discoveries that have revolutionized medicine and medical research.

6

Coming

Along at the

Right Time

Jonas Salk

At the end of World War II, prospects for the development of a polio vaccine appeared grim. The puzzle of the poliovirus still had many missing pieces, and polio researchers were haunted by memories of polio vaccine trials where things had gone very wrong.

In 1935, after experimenting with a formalin-inactivated vaccine that seemed to produce no adverse effects on twenty monkeys, Dr. Maurice Brodie, who was working at New York University under Dr. William H. Park, rashly decided to administer his vaccine to 3,000 children. At the same time, Dr. John Kolmer of Temple University in Philadelphia had concocted a live, attenuated vaccine, described by some as a "witch's brew."

Hundreds of children were given the two vaccines before their dangers became clear. Brodie's was ineffective and could cause severe allergic reactions, while Kolmer's vaccine had caused cases of polio, some of them fatal. The disastrous outcome of these premature human trials, due to mistakes, inadequate data, and the investigators' eagerness to outdo one another, dampened the scientific community's willingness to attempt human trials of a polio vaccine for many years.[1]

As he worked out the inactivation methods for his polio vaccine, the 1935 fiascos had to be present in the mind of Jonas Salk. Fortunately, he had other scientific precedents and developments to build upon, and he seized the opportunity provided by each one. Salk had come along at just the right time. Several scientific steppingstones were in place in the 1940s when he was ready to put his ideas about a polio vaccine into practice.

In 1935, the precursor to the National Foundation for Infantile Paralysis, the President's Birthday Ball Commission, had formed a scientific advisory committee to determine how to allocate research project grants. This committee's successor, the NFIP Committee on Scientific Research, began meeting in 1938. One of the first questions it laid on the table was: Is there more than one form of the poliovirus? Many scientists were convinced there was a single homogenous strain and had great difficulty believing in a family of polioviruses.

Although the members of the committee may not have been aware of it, an important hurdle to developing a vaccine had been overcome some years earlier. In 1931, two Australian researchers, Dr. Frank M. Burnet (later Sir Macfarlane Burnet) and Dame Jean Macnamara, had demonstrated that antigenic differences exist between at least two strains of poliovirus, and that immunity against one type will not confer protection against the other(s). Understanding that there were different strains of the virus was fundamental to attempts to vaccinate against the disease or develop tests to detect immunity.

In 1948, the NFIP finally set up the Committee on Typing to determine and classify, once and for all, the number of serotypes of the poliovirus. The Committee on Typing included several distinguished scientists and key players in the polio vaccine story. The typing program represented a milestone in the field of cooperative research; it involved several university laboratories working together and applying their talents toward a common goal.

Years later, a member of the NFIP's General Advisory Committee said that he considered the typing project "the greatest single piece of developmental research that the NFIP was to accomplish during the years of its existence," opening the way for all subsequent research. According to the polio researcher John Paul, "It was a major triumph for the NFIP to have engineered this cooperative endeavor among a highly individualistic group of research workers."[2]

Jonas Salk first became interested in poliomyelitis when he joined the typing program in 1948. Salk was thirty-three years old, a young and ambitious researcher and the newly appointed head of the Virus Research Lab at the University of Pittsburgh Medical School. His was one of four virus-typing laboratories that received NFIP support to test samples of the virus and type them according to strain—a long and tedious chore. When he accepted the job, the influenza virus, not the poliovirus, was his primary area of interest, but Salk welcomed the project as a means to expand and equip his new laboratory.

In 1949, David Bodian and his colleagues at Johns Hopkins University had described three basic immunological types of the poliovirus. His work was confirmed by the

Committee on Typing when it published its first results in 1951. Once it had been established that there were three and no more than three types of the poliovirus, researchers trying to develop a vaccine had at least identified their target. One vital steppingstone fell into place.

A trio of investigators in Boston was responsible for the next important breakthrough, which had repercussions well beyond the polio battlefield. It happened one day when Dr. Thomas Weller, a young associate working in the laboratory of Dr. John Enders at the Boston's Children's Hospital, produced too many tubes of culture medium for an experiment on chickenpox virus. Enders suggested he seed the extra tubes with some poliovirus in the laboratory freezer, which had been sent by the National Foundation. (Like many other virus research laboratories, Enders's lab received funding from American dimes.) To everyone's amazement, the poliovirus grew even though the medium contained no nervous-system tissues.[3]

In 1948, it was widely accepted among scientists that poliovirus would grow in a test tube only in medium containing nervous-system tissue. This was logical since the disease attacked the nervous system. In addition, experiments performed in 1936 by Albert Sabin and Peter Olitsky of the Rockefeller Institute seemed to confirm this theory. They were the first researchers to grow the poliovirus in test-tube cultures using a medium containing human embryonic nervous tissue. Because they were unable to cultivate it in any other human tissues, they erroneously concluded the poliovirus would multiply only in nerve cells. This represented a formidable hurdle to a potential vaccine, since nervous tissue injected in the body could cause fatal inflammatory reactions in the brain.[4]

The discovery in Boston disproved these commonly accepted tenets of polio research. The tissue culture method electrified the research community. It quickly became an invaluable technique for the practical study of polioviruses, paving the way for the inactivated and attenuated poliovirus vaccines. For the first time, researchers realized it would be possible to make large quantities of poliovirus for the development and production of a vaccine. In 1954, Enders, Weller, and colleague Dr. Frederick Robbins were awarded the Nobel Prize for their discovery.

Medical research is full of such seemingly lucky discoveries. Alexander Fleming discovered the first antibiotic after he forgot a culture dish in which antibiotic agents were able to kill colonies of bacteria. And yet, as Napoleon Bonaparte put it, "La chance sourit aux gros bataillons" (Luck smiles upon huge battalions). In science the huge battalions are patience, imagination, intuition, knowledge, and a keen sense of observation.

The good news for polio researchers was that their work would finally be less dependent on monkeys. Prior to tissue culture methods, polio research relied entirely on scientists using monkeys to isolate and identify the virus, a method that was complicated and expensive. Scientists had to infect individual monkeys, wait until they became sick, and then kill them to grind up their spinal columns and obtain the virus. One monkey would yield enough virus to make a few doses of vaccine. Procuring reliable supplies of monkeys, caring for them, making sure they were disease-free, and avoiding bites was a constant source of problems for researchers.

Rhesus monkeys, the type most commonly used in research, are considered sacred in the Hindu religion. They are incarnations of the monkey god Hanuman, also a fertility god and protector against whirlwinds.[5] The government of India put embargoes on monkey exports when it deemed the monkeys were being mistreated. Indeed, for several months in 1955, India imposed an embargo on monkey exports that meant the Connaught Laboratories were unable to produce the required amounts of virus culture fluids for the Canada-wide polio vaccination program.[6]

Obtaining sufficient quantities of virus for large-scale vaccine production using monkeys was worse than impractical. When he heard about the breakthrough in Boston, Jonas Salk was eager to equip his lab with the new production techniques, which would offer a way to complete the virus-typing project and work on a potential vaccine. He would still need monkeys to provide the tissue for the growth medium, but far fewer of them. He was thrilled when he could report that "the testicles of a single monkey can produce as many as 200 roller tubes of culture medium," according to Jane Smith.[7] By March 1953, the Virus Research Lab was using monkey kidney cells in their cultures, which seemed to provide even better results.

With these two achievements—the identification of the three strains and the fact that researchers could grow the virus in a test tube on non-nervous tissue—prospects for a polio vaccine brightened considerably. However, scientists still lacked a clear understanding of how polio infects the body. A generation of polio researchers had been convinced that the nose was the portal of entry of the disease to the body, reasoning that the virus traveled from the olfactory nerve directly into the brain and spinal cord.

Then, in the early 1950s, scientists isolated poliovirus in the blood, during the incubation period. Dr. Dorothy Millicent Horstmann of Yale University discovered that the poliovirus was present in the bloodstream before it attacked the nervous system and caused paralytic symptoms. This discovery was especially important for Salk and his approach. It meant that a killed-virus vaccine, the type he advocated, could be used to stimulate the production of antibodies in the blood and prevent the virus from entering the central nervous system. As John Paul writes, "In one fell swoop the problem of immunizing man had been rendered easier than was expected."

Salk had the good fortune to have studied virology with an eminent virologist, Dr. Thomas Francis, at the School of Public Health of the University of Michigan, where Salk had worked on an influenza vaccine. There he learned a great deal about virus inactivation and vaccine production, gaining invaluable experience in ways of developing and testing a vaccine. Francis was one of the few virologists, at that time, who thought it feasible to try and make a killed vaccine, and he thought it was worth trying.[8]

———

Today when people talk about the polio vaccines, they often make the distinction between IPV and OPV according to how the vaccines are administered (the IPV is injected while the OPV is given orally) or according to each vaccine's inventor (Salk, Sabin). In the 1940s and 1950s, while the public was clamoring for a vaccine and giving their dimes to make it a reality, polio researchers were divided between the dead-virus and live-virus vaccine approaches.

Jonas Salk belonged to the dead-virus school of thought and advocated a somewhat unorthodox vaccine based on completely inactivated, or killed, virus. Salk believed that the body could acquire immunity to polio without contracting the disease, through the injection of a killed virus whose presence in the blood would stimulate the production of antibodies. And, Salk thought, a killed-virus vaccine would generate higher levels of immunity to polio than a natural infection. When he began working on polio, one of his early ideas was to vaccinate chickens and cows with killed virus vaccine so the antibodies they produced would pass into milk and eggs for human consumption.[9]

By contrast, Albert Sabin was convinced that only a vaccine containing live, attenuated (weakened) virus, which imitates a natural infection, would confer lasting immunity. His approach followed classic principles of virology, the ones used by Edward Jenner and Louis Pasteur. He was older than Salk and more established in the virus research community. His reputation allowed him to enjoy more limelight than other scientists, such as Hilary Koprowski, who had begun working on an oral polio vaccine before Sabin.

Sabin had found low levels of polio antibodies in cow serum and hoped to identify a cow enterovirus similar to the human poliovirus. In such a way he could adopt Jenner's vaccine approach, since the cowpox virus elicited protective immunity against smallpox in humans without causing disease. Sabin did not find a bovine enterovirus close to the poliovirus, however, and turned definitively toward the other classic vaccine approach, developed by Pasteur, which consisted of attenuating the wild poliovirus.

When Salk first announced that he wanted to test his vaccine, Sabin was openly skeptical and voiced a long list of concerns. He was certain that ten to fifteen years of further study would be necessary before Salk's killed-virus vaccine would be practicable.

Several other research teams were working on a vaccine, but Jonas Salk was moving along faster than any of them. As his lab worked on the NFIP-funded Virus Typing Program, Salk experimented with methods for inactivating the virus and testing it. His vaccine preparation had to be potent enough to elicit an immune response, while being entirely safe. By the time the lab had completed the work for the typing program, in the spring of 1952, Salk felt ready to get beyond monkey testing and try his killed-virus preparation on humans. He was sure it was safe; now he wanted to see how effective it was.

Salk began small-scale, hush-hush trials of his vaccine in and around Pittsburgh. Only a few of the top people at the NFIP knew about them, and then only because they were funding them (Harry Weaver, Tom Rivers, Basil O'Connor); the NFIP money was the lifeblood of the struggle to defeat polio.

Next, he asked for permission to administer the vaccine and monitor blood antibody levels among children and inmates in two institutions not far from Pittsburgh: the Polk State School, a center for retarded male children and adults, and the Watson Home for Crippled Children. At the Watson Home, Salk set out to prove that his killed-virus vaccine produced higher levels of immunity than a natural infection. Lorraine Friedman, Salk's assistant, accompanied him on all his visits. She devised a meticulous system to record vaccination dates and blood test results on index cards.

In the mid-twentieth century, conducting clinical trials in prisons, orphanages, and homes for the mentally retarded was common practice. It gave researchers access to volunteers in a single geographic location, whose age, gender, and general health were documented. Furthermore, the individuals were certain to be present at each visit included in the trial protocol. The various prototypes of live and inactivated polio vaccines were first tested under such conditions, before being tested in large-scale trials. Rules concerning informed consent were less strict than at the end of the twentieth century.

Salk changed variables, formulations, and adjuvants, determined to figure out which vaccine formulation worked best. He went home one day and vaccinated his three sons in the kitchen. He also tried the vaccine on members of his laboratory. In the spring of 1953, he conducted a "family trial" in which some 600 people took part, and by the fall approximately 700 people had been inoculated with a vaccine produced by his lab.[10]

These small trials, which required giving shots, drawing blood samples, testing and recording antibody levels, and keeping careful records, involved a tremendous amount of work. Salk gave people the impression that he was everywhere at once, but behind the scenes many people were holding down the fort back at the Virus Research Laboratory, which had become something of a poliovirus production plant. As one indicator of its activity, in early 1953, the lab, which had a full-time staff of twenty-five in addition to volunteers and grad students, ordered weekly shipments of one thousand white mice and fifty monkeys.

As the summer approached, and with it, the dread of another polio season, the urgency of the hunt pressed upon Salk and his team. The need to develop a vaccine quickly never left their minds for long. The Virus Research Laboratory in Pittsburgh was housed alongside the Municipal Hospital where, in the summer of 1953, four hundred new patients were admitted to the polio ward.

Salk felt pressure from all sides: from the NFIP, which was giving premature hints to the American public that a vaccine was just around the corner; from the media; and from his fellow scientists, many of whom publicly cast doubt on his vaccine. He also felt pressure from anxious parents, who put blind faith in science.

It had become clear that a national field trial was needed in order to test the safety and efficacy of the Salk polio vaccine; debate raged over how to organize it and who would oversee it. The NFIP assumed it would retain control, while the U.S. government's Public Health Service's Communicable Disease Center (the predecessor to the Centers for

Disease Control) felt most suited to do the job.[11] Meanwhile, many members of the scientific community contested both the wisdom of the trial and the plans to administer it. In testimony before Congress, Albert Sabin, who had become their chief spokesman, stated his strong opposition to the trial, hoping to delay a national test until his own vaccine was ready.

Tensions ran high in the months leading up to the decisions on if, when, and how to stage a field trial. Finally it was decided: Dr. Thomas Francis, director of the University of Michigan's School of Health, would oversee the largest and most highly publicized field trial ever attempted. Everyone agreed that the integrity of a study he supervised would be beyond reproach.

Dr. Francis accepted this daunting, extremely complex task, but he set the conditions. Chief among them was that he alone would design and retain full control over the trial, and his evaluation would focus on a double-blind field trial, with half the children given an inert placebo as a control. Salk and the NFIP would have to wait along with the rest of the world to hear the results.

In late January 1954, Thomas Francis drafted the terms on which he would supervise the trial. Now the question was, could it possibly be organized before the next polio season began?

7

Behind the

Scenes

Toronto, Canada, 1954

March 29, 1954. The Canadian edition of *Time* is hot off the press, and Toronto's renowned Connaught Laboratories are featured in this issue's cover story. Canada has just endured its worst polio epidemic the previous year. *Time*'s cover asks the question on everyone's lips: "Polio Fighter Salk: Is This the Year?"

Across North America, families are fretting over whether their children will be able to go to the local swimming pool or to summer camp in a few months' time. The public is longing for news of substance about a vaccine that has been the subject of hopes, promises, and controversy—not to mention extraordinary press coverage—over the preceding months and years.

Will the vaccine work? How soon will the field trial begin? From Jonas Salk to the NFIP president Basil O'Connor to Mrs. Olveta Culp Hobby, the U.S. Secretary of Health, Education and Welfare, no one knows. Not even the medical journalists at *Time*. There was still great uncertainty about the polio vaccine.

Jonas Salk is portrayed in his lab coat on the cover of *Time*. Next to him is the artist's collage of virus particles, abandoned leg splints, crutches, and a row of vaccine-filled syringes. Little children are running, jumping, and roller skating around the letters T-I-M-E. On page 60, the Medicine section opens with a simple title: "Closing in on Polio" where it explains that "Dr. Salk's laboratories could not produce more than a fraction of the hundreds of gallons of vaccine needed" for a massive field trial. Then it describes Toronto's Connaught Laboratories, today sanofi-aventis, which provided the critical bulk fluids for making the vaccine.

Time explains how polio viral fluids, the basis of any vaccine, are made. The description, which leaves nothing to the imagination, provides a definition of tissue culture, explaining how tiny bits of monkey kidneys are suspended in nutrients to provide the ideal environment in which to grow the poliovirus.

> The University of Toronto's Connaught Medical Research Laboratories use 60 to 65 monkeys in a single morning. Each is deeply anesthetized with ether. In a couple of minutes a skilled surgeon removes the kidneys. Then the monkey is killed with an overdose of ether. Patient technicians cut the kidneys into tiny pieces with nail scissors. The bits of tissue go into big glass bottles with a pink solution known by its formula designation: No. 199. Hundreds of bottles are rocked gently for six days in an incubator, and kidney cells grow in the fluid as though they were still in the living animal.
>
> In a room with the safety rules and precautions of a radioisotope laboratory, 2 cc. of fluid containing live poliovirus are added as a seed stock to each quart of

tissue fluid. Back to the rocker go the bottles. The virus multiplies a thousand-fold in the kidney cells, and after about four days the potentially deadly crop is ready for harvest. It is chilled in $2^1/_2$ gal. bottles for trucking from Toronto to Eli Lilly & Co. and to Parke, Davis.[1]

The article mentions two Connaught discoveries that were crucial to the large-scale production and success of Jonas Salk's polio vaccine: Medium 199, the synthetic growth medium in which liters and liters of poliovirus could be grown safely, and the "Toronto Method" of rocking bottles, invented and perfected by Connaught's Dr. Leone Norwood Farrell. Without these two innovations, the largest field trial in history, involving nearly two million children, would not have been possible.

———

The National Foundation for Infantile Paralysis (later known as the March of Dimes) first took an interest in Toronto's research capacities some fourteen years earlier when, in 1940, it gave Connaught Laboratories a $9,200 grant to fund polio field studies. It renewed these grants through 1943, when polio research had to take a back seat as the laboratories focused on supplying the typhus vaccine to the Canadian armed forces.

Then, in the summer of 1947, Andrew J. Rhodes, a native of Scotland and an internationally recognized virologist and polio authority, arrived in Toronto. He had been recruited by Connaught's Dr. Robert Defries. He was to head Connaught's polio research efforts from 1947 to 1953 and, in 1948–1949, to direct the investigation of a polio epidemic among Canadian Eskimos, where he was able to study the transmission of the virus in an isolated community.

Connaught's monkey-housing facilities were expanded

in accordance with NFIP requirements, as the public grew increasingly desperate over polio and the NFIP was reconsidering its approach to funding research. The NFIP was especially interested in working with Connaught, a noncommercial, university-based institution. Founded in 1914 as part of the University of Toronto, Connaught had established a reputation in vaccine development and production. Its highly qualified scientific staff included many bright, skillful women scientists.

In 1947, the NFIP was ready to finance a comprehensive polio research program at Connaught that would take advantage of Connaught's capacity for a large monkey colony. Connaught was one of the few laboratories in North America with facilities that could accommodate a large number of monkeys.

Rhodes began experimenting with ways to grow the poliovirus in test tubes; he visited Dr. John Enders's laboratory in Boston to learn his team's culturing techniques. In May 1951, the NFIP honored Rhodes by asking him to sit on their newly established Committee on Immunization, whose members were all leading figures in polio research.[2] In May 1952, Harry Weaver, the NFIP's research director, asked the Connaught Laboratories to conduct a pilot project on producing the virus in huge quantities. The NFIP agreed to fund the expansion of Rhodes's program, which would require six hundred monkeys in addition to new equipment and more staff. With a final NFIP grant of $104,500, polio research grants accounted for half of all outside grants to Connaught for that year.

Frank Shimada, a Connaught retiree who started out inoculating monkeys at Connaught when he joined the company in 1949, worked alongside Dr. Rhodes as one of his principal technicians. The structure and ambience at Connaught and the University of Toronto's School of Hygiene, he says, allowed cross-fertilization of expertise to successfully launch large-scale polio vaccine production.

"For example, the synthetic Medium 199 so critical to produce large volumes of poliovirus fluid was developed by a research group studying cell metabolism in tissue culture for cancer research, while the bacterial vaccine group provided us with large 'Povitsky' flasks used for diphtheria vaccine production," says Frank.[3]

The bottles used for diphtheria culture turned out to be about the right size to use on the rocking machines. "This sharing of knowledge was vital in saving time in the race to meet the international demand for polio vaccine," Frank adds.

The pilot project experimented with growing the virus in various solutions and ever larger containers. It demonstrated that monkey kidneys were the organ of choice for viral cultures; it became clear later that kidneys are essentially "dirty" organs that bring their own set of problems, notably the need to ensure that tissue cultures are free of other viruses before the poliovirus can be introduced.[4]

When NFIP organizers began to prepare for the field trial of the Salk vaccine, they realized they needed a massive mobilization of people and materials in a short amount of time. The logistics were mind-boggling—to take just one example, locating 1,200,000 sterile needles, more than could be found anywhere in the United States, seemed an insurmountable problem.[5] One of the most pressing needs was, of course, sufficient quantities of the Salk vaccine, which takes more than one year to produce from start to finish.

The Connaught scientists who created Medium 199 initially called it *Mixture* #199 because it corresponded to the 199th attempt to combine sixty ingredients.[6] Two scientists in Dr. Raymond Parker's laboratory had developed the mixture for cancer research. Dr. Parker was an eminent investigator in the field of tissue culture who had studied for nine years at the Rockefeller Institute in New York with the French biologist Dr. Alexis Carrel, widely regarded as the father of *in vitro* tissue culture—growing cells outside of the body.

This synthetic growth medium supported chick embryo cells for an average of thirty-three days. Because it was harmless—it contained no animal serum or other proteins—it was superbly suited to the preparation of a vaccine for use in humans. In the early 1950s, Connaught researchers published a series of papers showing that Medium 199 supported the growth of all three types of poliovirus.

Jonas Salk phoned Dr. Parker and asked for a small supply of the formula so he could produce his own. Soon he reported a preliminary series of inoculations with a vaccine prepared from virus culture fluids using monkey kidney cells grown on Medium 199.[7] Harmless Medium 199 solution would also be used as a placebo during the field trial, given in place of the vaccine to all the young Polio Pioneers who served as controls. On a broader scale, in the words of Dr. Andrew Rhodes, "Mixture 199 played a major role in the modern era of progress in the laboratory study of viruses in cell cultures."[8]

As historian Christopher Rutty points out, it is also the story of a friendship between two biochemists who met at Connaught. Dr. Arthur E. Franklin, who joined Rhodes's polio group in June 1951, formed a friendship with Dr. Joseph F. Morgan in Parker's laboratory and from him learned about Medium 199, which Morgan had developed with Helen J. Morton. Franklin tried it and, to his delight and surprise, discovered it was perfect for cultivating the poliovirus. Franklin recounted that when Rhodes, his research director, first learned about the results with Medium 199, he jumped up on a chair and cheered in an uncharacteristic display of emotion.[9]

In addition to providing the right growth medium, Connaught researchers also developed methods to grow the poliovirus in large quantities. In particular, Dr. Leone Norwood Farrell, a specialist in mycology, the science of fungi, helped launch the era of mass-produced vaccines with her invention of a system to rock bottles of culture fluids. She first devised the method in 1945 for the production of a whooping cough (pertussis) vaccine.

What soon became known as the "Toronto Method" consisted of strapping bottles filled with culture fluids onto large boards that were stacked much like trays of cookies cooling on a bakery cart. The boards were rocked mechanically, producing a gentle motion that exposed the fluids in the bottles to a "greater depth of nutrient."[10]

In June 1953, the NFIP made its first request for 420 liters of fluids containing types 1, 2, and 3 of the poliovirus. By August, the amount had increased to 2,000 liters, so that Connaught's target was to supply 186 liters every two weeks. In all, the Connaught Laboratories produced a total of 5,521 liters of fluid, using more than 7,000 monkeys.[11] They provided nearly all the poliomyelitis virus fluids from which the vaccines used in the 1954 field trials were made. In a 1954 letter to Dr. Defries, Jonas Salk described this as "a Herculean task."[12]

Nearly fifty years later, people still like to tell the story of how the viral fluids produced at Connaught sloshed around in the back of a station wagon as it traveled across the Canadian border to two pharmaceutical houses: Parke-Davis in Detroit, and Eli Lilly in Indianapolis. The fluids were then inactivated and transformed into a vaccine.

Says Frank Shimada, "Connaught's expertise mandated that we would provide the large volumes of poliovirus fluid which allowed U.S. pharmaceutical companies to develop virus inactivation processes simultaneously." He explains that this spirit of international cooperation between companies, as well as with the government testing and regulatory agencies, provided the impetus to complete the mission successfully.

Relations between the NFIP and the Connaught Laboratories were carefully managed and kept quiet. Beyond the inner circle of those involved, the story of the development of the polio vaccine by staff from Connaught was not widely known.

Officials at the NFIP were concerned about the public's reaction if people found out that U.S. dimes were being sent north of the border to fund research. In 1949, Dr. Defries wrote to the president of the University of Toronto, Sidney Smith, to explain why funding from the National Foundation should not be publicized: "As the [directors of the] Foundation are embarrassed by making grants for this work in the University of Toronto from the campaign funds of the March of Dimes in the United States, I understand that they would appreciate no public announcement of these grants."[13]

Jonas Salk visited Toronto a number of times and the Connaught staff traveled to Pittsburgh to observe operations in Salk's laboratory, especially vaccine testing. Says Frank Shimada, "By the time Salk had done his initial trials, he had in his lab doctors learning developing techniques from Australia and doctors from South Africa and Germany. These representatives returned to their countries to complete their vaccine projects—truly an international effort."

Although Connaught's role was to supply bulk fluids to be used in making the vaccine, Dr. Defries wanted his team to learn all aspects of vaccine production. He wanted the lab to be ready. In April 1955, a mass polio vaccination program was launched to immunize 500,000 children across Canada, using vaccine manufactured at Connaught.

The U.S. and Canadian approaches to polio research and

the efforts to develop a vaccine could not have been more different. South of the Canadian border, the U.S. federal government spent very little on polio research (in 1953, a total of $72,000 compared to $2 million spent by the NFIP).[14] Government officials were content to let a private charity fund research, especially basic research. They also were content to have the NFIP provide assistance to polio victims and their families and dispense training and information to medical personnel.

Although the federal government would decide whether or not to license the Salk vaccine—and any other polio vaccines for commercial manufacture—it took a hands-off approach to research, confident that medical care and drug development were best left up to free enterprise, without undue interference from the government. When the time came to decide whether or not to license the Salk vaccine, government officials at the U.S. Laboratory of Biologics Control, a subdivision of the National Institutes of Health (NIH), had much to learn about polio.

The scientists discovered it was no easy task to teach bureaucrats about the intricacies and epidemiology of a viral disease. Said Dr. Tom Rivers, a renowned immunologist and one of the core group of scientists who advised the NFIP from the outset: "The Public Health Service would eventually have to license the vaccine, and nobody knew anything about polio. . . . We had an awful time teaching them about polio."[15] As part of his education, William Workman, director of the Laboratory of Biologics Control, visited Connaught Laboratories in 1953 to study the procedures for growing poliovirus in tissue culture.

From a Canadian perspective, the state and federal governments were notably absent from the polio story in the United States, setting the stage for tragic consequences. The creation and development of the NFIP, a private charity, precluded the involvement of the government, while the opposite was true in Canada. The Canadian Foundation for Poliomyelitis, or CFP, was founded in 1948 to be built on the American model, but the methods, ideas, and publicity that were so successful in the United States could not easily be transplanted to Canada.[16]

On October 17, 1955, Dr. Defries was awarded the prestigious Albert Lasker Award from the American Public Health Association in recognition of his own role and Connaught's contribution to the development of the Salk vaccine. The award was presented by former U.S. President Harry Truman.

Looking back on that era, Frank Shimada, a Connaught employee from 1949 to 1988, says, "Today you couldn't do half of what we did back then. I suppose we were making up the rules as we went along. . . . It was a race against time. The idea was to save children. By today's standards we were idealistic and perhaps romantic, but we did succeed!"

8

The Largest

Medical

Experiment

in History

United States, 1954

McLean, Virginia, April 26, 1954. Six-year-old Randy Kerr stepped up to receive an injection of the Salk polio vaccine. He was the first Polio Pioneer to participate in the Francis Field Trial, the largest medical experiment in history. The trial's design, the result of protracted and lively debate among the NFIP and scientists, was intended to assess the safety and efficacy of the killed-virus vaccine. The families of nearly two million children volunteered for them to take part in the trial. These Polio Pioneers from 217 health districts across forty-four states in the United States were enrolled in the trial, in addition to children in Finland and in forty-six health districts in Canada.

Parental consent was of course necessary for every Polio Pioneer. In a stroke of genius, NFIP staff came up with the idea of calling the permission slip parents had to sign a "request" form rather than a consent form. Such linguistic dexterity made the children enrolled in the trial not guinea pigs, but part of a privileged group. Indeed, many parents saw it this way. No one, from the doctors giving the shots to the record keepers and administrators, knew what was in the syringes, placebo or the "real stuff," a vaccine against all three strains of polio. This was what scientists call a double-blind trial.

At the University of Michigan in Ann Arbor, the specially built Poliomyelitis Vaccine Evaluation Center would centralize the records concerning all the first- to third-graders enrolled in the trial: 1.2 million children served as a control group (receiving no vaccination), while more than 650,000 received injections. Roughly 440,000 received one or more injections of a vaccine, and about 210,000 children received a placebo, consisting of harmless Medium 199. Children in the control group were observed to see if any contracted polio.

The Polio Pioneers were watched closely, since only about 10 percent of individuals who are infected by the poliovirus develop any identifiable symptoms of the disease. If the number of cases among the unvaccinated group was significantly higher than among children who had received the vaccine, this would provide evidence that the vaccine worked.

An estimated 150,000 to 300,000 volunteers contributed their time and energy during the trial: doctors, nurses, school principals, teachers, and family members came to distribute lollipops and Polio Pioneer buttons. Basil O'Connor, director of the NFIP, insisted on using volunteers rather than paid employees, reasoning that they would work for free and with a great sense of commitment.[1] Because these mostly local NFIP volunteers were known and trusted by their communities, they formed an instant network of field trial supporters—a result similar to naming local postmasters to be chairmen of the Birthday Balls, the forerunners to the March of Dimes fund-raising campaigns.

The logistical details had to be worked out with great speed; with the arrival of warm weather and the beginning of a new polio season, it would be impossible to tell which children developed antibodies in response to the vaccine and which had been exposed naturally to the poliovirus. The planned vaccination of children in certain southern states had to be dropped because the polio season had already begun in these warmer climates. To make up for the dropped states and maintain the planned size of the trial, the organizers added forty-six local Canadian health districts and two areas in Finland.

——

Right up to the eve of the opening of the Francis Field Trial, there was still uncertainty among the scientists and administrators as to whether or not the trial would go ahead. One day before the first Polio Pioneer was immunized, the NFIP Vaccine Advisory Committee was still in intense discussions about what to do. Among the scientists, the medical profession, and organizers, there were lingering fears, for example, that the vaccine might actually cause polio. The 1935 vaccine trial attempts by Maurice Brodie and John Kolmer, which had ended in fiascos, still haunted them.

Jonas Salk was convinced that his vaccine was safe and would prevent polio. Indeed, for Salk, it was not a specific vaccine formulation that was on trial as much as his general theory of immunization—a theory holding that a vaccine based on killed (or inactivated) virus would stimulate antibody production in the bloodstream and bring protection against polio. Salk the immunologist had confidence in a mathematical model he developed to determine the precise relationship between the amount of formalin used for inactivation, the concentration of the poliovirus, and the length of time the formalin had to stay in contact with the virus to safely inactivate it. He trusted a mathematical formula to ensure that the vaccine contained no pathogenic virus.

Salk's ideas were new; they clashed with those of older scientists and with the traditional approach to vaccines based on the smallpox model. According to the conventional model, a vaccine should be made from an attenuated (weakened), living virus that would provoke a natural but mildly immunizing infection without causing disease. Not surprisingly, the advocates of the two approaches—killed vaccine versus attenuated vaccine—each thought the other's vaccine was dangerous and entailed taking unnecessary risks.

Pragmatic souls such as Basil O'Connor, the forceful director of the NFIP, saw the polio problem from a different perspective. O'Connor weighed the risks associated with the Salk vaccine against those that loomed ahead with the summer and a new polio season. Salk was watching to see whether his ideas, not his specific vaccine formulation, would work, while O'Connor reasoned that even a mediocre vaccine offering protection to some people would begin to save lives; using it now was better than waiting for a perfect vaccine that might not be available for years.

Publicity surrounding the trial reached a peak in early April 1954 and marked an open season for settling old scores with O'Connor, Salk, and the NFIP. Researchers who were working on other vaccines, notably Albert Sabin, who was on the way to developing an attenuated oral vaccine, were openly critical. Some people tried to sabotage the field trial by using scare tactics aimed at parents. Walter Winchell, a radio show host and syndicated columnist, spread rumors that the NFIP had a stock of little white coffins for the children who would die as a result of their involvement in the trial.[2]

Organizations such as the American Medical Association voiced fears that immunization clinics would usher in the dreaded specter of socialized medicine. In addition, the months of vaccine administration during the trial coincided with national broadcasts of hearings led by Senator Joseph McCarthy, which created a backdrop of insecurity about another disease: the contagion of communism.

All this was, however, background noise for most parents. The public pressure in favor of the trial and parents' willingness to have their children take part prevailed. In some schools, 90 percent of eligible children returned their request-to-participate forms. By the end of June, the participants in the field trial had received the last of their shots. All the registers were sent to Ann Arbor, where the data would be interpreted, a formidable task that would take no less than nine months. A Gallup poll conducted on May 31, 1954, revealed that more Americans knew about the polio field trial than knew the name of their country's president.[3]

––––

Ann Arbor, Michigan, April 12, 1955. This was the day on which the results of the Francis Field Trial were announced. It coincided with the tenth anniversary of the death of Franklin Roosevelt, the world's most famous polio victim, and marked the climax in the long search for a polio vaccine, the culmination of decades of scientific research, years of effort, and millions of dollars from the March of Dimes funds.

The world's ears and eyes were fixed on Rackham Hall on the University of Michigan campus where the Vaccine Evaluation Center was located. The public had been waiting for confirmation that the Salk vaccine worked, and now that the announcement was just minutes away, the more than one hundred journalists who had flocked to the third floor of Rackham Hall were burning to know the results. Reporters had come from across the United States as well as Canada, France, and beyond. There were even television camera crews, although TV news was still something of a novelty in 1955.

Two conferences had been planned: one in a small auditorium for the press upstairs, and, in the large auditorium on the main floor, a scientific meeting where Dr. Thomas Francis would unveil his report at 10:20 A.M. The reporters who were packed into the press room had been told they would receive a press packet at 9:10 A.M. but were not allowed to release anything until Dr. Francis began speaking. When they still had nothing at 9:15, they began to lie in wait opposite the elevator doors. When the doors opened, the journalists mobbed the hand cart carrying the report, grabbing copies. The University of Michigan press secretary was forced to stand on a table and toss out reports to the hungry crowd. The next day's issue of the *Detroit News* described the scene:

> The press releases were in boxes on a hand truck. To avoid a crush, public relations men from the university began throwing the releases into the crowd. But still, hands grabbed at the boxes. In the next few seconds, pandemonium prevailed. Then there was a dash for the couple of dozen typewriters in the press room and for a battery of telephones.[4]

The journalists greedily scanned the report and press release, which went straight to the point: "The vaccine works. It is safe, effective and potent." They shouted to each other, "It works! It works!" Then they raced to file their stories.

People in the scientific meeting downstairs were unaware of the mayhem in the press room. Most of the scientists who received NFIP funding were in the auditorium,
including Salk's rival and critic, Albert Sabin. The NFIP staff
had turned out in force. The Vaccine Evaluation Center
team, which had worked so diligently over the previous nine
months to produce the Francis Report; the researchers from
Jonas Salk's lab; Salk's wife, Donna, and their three sons;
and representatives of the Watson Home for Crippled Children where Salk had conducted preliminary trials of his
vaccine, were all present.

The presidents of the six companies that had been producing polio vaccine also wanted to be present when the
results were announced. Dr. Robert Defries, traveling with
Dr. G.D.W. Cameron, Canadian deputy minister of health,
had made the trip from Connaught Laboratories in Toronto.
In Toronto, the Connaught staff, busy preparing vaccine for
the Canadian field trial, would watch a broadcast with a
digest of the Francis Report from 6 to 7 P.M. at the King
Edward Hotel. The drug company Eli Lilly had paid for the
closed-circuit broadcast to be transmitted to physicians in
sixty-one cities in the United States and Canada.

Ever since the beginning of the Francis Field Trial, people
had speculated about the efficacy of the vaccine. Many sur-
mised that organizers knew the vaccine worked, or they
would not have given it to nearly two million children, but
this assumption was mistaken. No one knew whether it
worked. Even Jonas Salk, whose confidence in the safety of
his vaccine had never wavered, had no idea as to how effective it would be. Thomas Francis, who had kept the first
results a closely guarded secret throughout those months,
had told Salk over breakfast, just prior to the announcement,
that his report would be favorable.

In the auditorium of Rackham Hall, Thomas Francis

presented his findings, speaking for over ninety minutes, illustrating his remarks with charts and graphs. The results were unequivocal: The Salk vaccine was safe and had protected the children who took it. The figures varied, depending on the manufacturer and the strain of the virus (type 1, 2, or 3). When groups of vaccinated children were compared to unvaccinated groups, the vaccine turned out to be 60–70 percent effective against type 1 polio and over 90 percent effective against types 2 and 3. It was 94 percent effective against bulbar polio, the frightening form that impaired breathing and required patients to live in an iron lung.[5]

Headlines the next day cried victory over the disease in no uncertain terms: "Salk's Vaccine Does the Job against Polio" (*Chicago Daily News*); "Salk Polio Vaccine Proves Success—Millions Will Be Immunized Soon" (*New York Times*). The vaccine was immediately licensed for distribution and crates marked "polio vaccine/ RUSH" began to leave vaccine manufacturers' warehouses.

Many people whose eyes were focused on Ann Arbor had a stake in the largest medical experiment in history. The parents of the Polio Pioneers rejoiced in having allowed their misgivings about the vaccine to be overcome. Hollywood celebrities such as Eddy Cantor and Helen Hayes greeted the news as enthusiastically as the hundreds of thousands of NFIP volunteers and donors who had channeled their terror of polio into constructive action and contributions to the March of Dimes.

The announcement that the Salk vaccine worked was a landmark in twentieth-century history, some of the best news ever to make the news and was indelibly burned in people's memories, like Neil Armstrong taking man's first steps on the moon on July 21, 1969. Salk felt gratified and relieved, especially after the criticism he had endured at the hands of his peers in the scientific community. After years

> The prestigious scientific journal *Nature* hailed the development of the first polio vaccine as one of the top-five scientific achievements of the twentieth century.
>
> "Some milestones in history are eagerly anticipated, much celebrated, and repeatedly recalled: the first polio vaccine, the first landing on the Moon, and the first non-stop transatlantic flight are good examples."
> —Vaclav Smil, Millennium Essay, *Nature*, September 30, 1999.

of anxiety and defending his ideas, his work had paid off and his theories had been vindicated. Overnight he became an international hero, the focus of a deluge of phone calls, letters, donations, and more attention than he ever dreamed possible. From then on it would be hard for him to concentrate on research, amidst all the publicity, requests for interviews, offers of honorary degrees, and speaking opportunities.

So much fame was hard to manage. As journalist Edward Murrow told Jonas Salk, something tragic had happened that day: he had lost his anonymity. And the more media attention he received, the more his fellow scientists mistrusted and resented him.

Many in the scientific community were horrified by the "forces of publicity and sensationalism" surrounding the announcement and the fact that the results were not presented first at the meeting of "an important scientific society." Due to the massive media attention, the public swiftly concluded that the Salk vaccine was perfect and that polio had been conquered. In fact, the vaccine needed to be improved and the disease was far from conquered.

The reaction of John Paul, a researcher who was experimenting with a live-virus vaccine at Yale, is probably characteristic of what many scientists felt. In his authoritative work, *A History of Poliomyelitis*, he writes: "The circumstances under which the report was released proved to be a temporary disaster for the reputation of American science. . . . One witness described the performance as being set to the tune of 'the rockets red glare and flashbulbs bursting in air.' [The Evaluation Center's work] did not deserve to be so cheapened by the outburst that ensued."[6]

Once the excitement of April 12 had settled down, the next challenge was to make the shift from research operation to mass production. How would the vaccine actually reach some 150 million people? The U.S. public health authorities had not dealt with important, predictable issues such as pricing, whether state or federal bodies would bear the cost of immunization, and who should have priority for limited supplies of polio vaccine. HEW secretary Olveta Culp Hobby had accorded the license to manufacture the vaccine without making provisions for safety controls or a distribution plan. During the field trial, each batch of vaccine had undergone three independent sets of controls to ensure it was safe and contained no live virus. Now that the trial was over, government officials performed only random checks, leaving each manufacturer responsible for its own controls.

On April 22, Jonas Salk received a special citation at the White House, presented by President Dwight Eisenhower. Two days later, and only twelve days after the euphoria in Ann Arbor, the bubble suddenly burst. Six cases of polio were reported in Chicago and California among children who had received vaccine made by the Cutter Laboratories in Berkeley. More reports followed, including secondary cases among parents of children who had been vaccinated. On April 27, the Cutter vaccine was pulled off the market. Confusion and crisis ensued, with public health officials and scientists accusing one another of bungling and mismanagement. On May 7, Leonard Scheele, the surgeon general, suspended all vaccine programs across the country. The next day he declared a national ban on polio vaccine manufacturing and put an embargo on vaccine exports.

What had happened? Eventually, it became clear that all the cases of polio could be traced to one manufacturer. Some lots of Cutter vaccine contained living virus, in clumps of virus that had escaped the inactivation process; insufficient controls had not detected the danger. In the final assessment, a total of 204 vaccine-associated cases of polio had occurred, 79 among vaccinated children and 105 among family contacts of these children. There were eleven deaths. After 1955, the CDC did not record a single case of polio linked to the Salk vaccine in the United States.

Two positive developments came out of this tragedy. First, the committees of experts created during the crisis concluded that the Mahoney type 1 polio strain was too virulent and needed to be replaced by a less virulent strain in preparing the vaccine. Second, this incident greatly contributed to the formation of a permanent surveillance unit at the Centers of Disease Control (CDC) to monitor outbreaks of disease.[7] The CDC's work following the Cutter crisis helped establish its role in the study and control of epidemics.

At the same time, north of the border, every batch of vaccine produced at Connaught (the only polio vaccine production site in Canada) was checked by the Connaught Laboratories and by the government's Laboratory of Hygiene. Nearly half a million Canadians had already received a dose of vaccine. There were no reports of vaccine-related paralysis, but in light of the U.S. deaths caused by the Cutter vaccine, Paul Martin Sr. faced one of his most difficult decisions as the Canadian minister of national health and welfare: whether or not to continue the country's vaccination program. He had personal experience with the disease, having contracted polio in 1907 as a child. His son, Paul Martin Jr., who would one day become the Canadian prime minister, was also stricken with polio when he was eight years old.

After much soul-searching, on May 8, the day after the surgeon general had called off the U.S. program, Paul Martin Sr. announced the polio vaccination program would continue in Canada. Events in Canada helped salvage the reputation of the Salk vaccine and meant a great deal to Jonas Salk. As Robert Defries would write later, "The decision in Canada to continue the program had a stabilizing effect on official and public opinion in the United States."[8]

In Denmark, the National Serum Institute produced its own vaccine using techniques based on what Preben and Herdis von Magnus had learned in March 1953 when they visited Salk's laboratory. To make up for a lack of inactivated virus, the Danish institute administered the vaccine in subcutaneous injections, which required smaller doses of vaccine than intramuscular injections. As was the case in Canada, the Danish immunization program continued without a hitch.

In the United States, immunization with the Salk vaccine resumed in June 1955 and had an immediate impact: the incidence of polio fell from 13.9 per 100,000 people in 1954 to 0.5 per 100,000 in 1961. The remaining epidemic outbreaks essentially occurred in the poorest urban populations where some people were not vaccinated. The same trend was observed in Canada and Denmark.

The injectable inactivated vaccine had clearly proven its effectiveness. Now the challenge was to produce it in large enough quantities so that the vaccine would be available in all countries where immunization was offered. As for the oral vaccine, made using live, attenuated virus, at the end of the 1950s it was still in the development phase.

9

The Race

for an Oral

Vaccine

United States, 1950–1960

On February 27, 1950, an eight-year-old boy from Letchworth Village, New York, received a prototype of the oral polio vaccine Hilary Koprowski had developed using the live, weakened (attenuated) virus. The boy suffered no side effects and Koprowski enlarged his experiment to include nineteen other children.

At the time Koprowski was a scientist at Lederle Laboratories, a fast-growing pharmaceutical company. Since 1948 he had been working on a viral attenuation process:

> A spinal cord suspension infected with Brockman's virus was adapted through successive passages on the brains of Swiss albino mice [. . .]. By the seventh passage, the vaccine was safe; it could be injected without harm to the monkey brains. The virus made for mice then underwent passages on rats. After one to three passages, the vaccine was ready.[1]

Later Koprowski realized that this strain, which he believed to be type 1, the most common type, was actually type 2. He renamed it TN. As he would write forty-five years later, "We had taken the path that would lead us to polio eradication."

———

His results were excellent. The virus was found in the stools of everyone who received the vaccine, which indicated it had reproduced in their digestive systems and triggered the production of antibodies. When the immunized children received the vaccine a second time, they were not reinfected, evidence that they were protected. The findings were so spectacular that when Koprowski presented them to a meeting of the NFIP's Immunization Committee, the committee members greeted them with skepticism.

All of these events took place four years before the Francis Field Trial of the Salk vaccine, but the oral polio vaccine would not be ready for use until five years after the injectable vaccine reached the market.

Strong teams were competing to make an oral polio vaccine, including one led by Albert Sabin of the Children's Hospital Research Foundation in Cincinnati as well as the one led by Hilary Koprowski of the Wistar Institute in Philadelphia, which he joined in 1957. Obtaining attenuated viral strains was an arduous task, which Koprowski likened to Hercules cleaning the Augean stables. Koprowski wrote that while his chore was less difficult, it was much more time-consuming because the same process had to be repeated again and again.

In 1951, Koprowski tested a prototype of the vaccine containing attenuated strains of types 1 and 2 on a group of sixty-one children in Sonoma State Home, an institute for mentally retarded children. The type 1 strains had been attenuated by twenty-seven passages inoculated intraspinally in mice. Later, cell cultures would be used for virus attenuation.[2]

Herald Cox, who first hired Koprowski at Lederle, had a falling-out with him in 1952 and became one of his rivals. According to Roger Vaughan, Lederle invested an estimated $13 million in the development of a live attenuated polio vaccine.

Albert Sabin, who was also working on live attenuated strains, paid a visit to Koprowski's lab at Lederle. In the words of Koprowski, the purpose of Sabin's visit was "to bury the hatchet and exchange samples of viruses. So I sent him some of my samples. But I never received any of his samples from him."

Maurice Hilleman, a major figure in vaccine research in America and director of the Merck Institute for Therapeutic Research, explains tersely that Sabin, "a self-pronounced genius, went in and took over Cox's and Koprowski's ideas."[3] According to John Paul, Koprowski would later complain that the polio vaccine he had discovered became known as the Sabin vaccine.

Many people were surprised at the viciousness of the disputes surrounding the discovery of the AIDS virus in the late 1980s. Those controversies were, however, no more characterized by dissension than the controversies surrounding research to develop a polio vaccine. In addition, they were confined to competition between two teams: Robert Gallo's team at the National Institutes of Health, and a team of Parisian physicians and virologists working with Luc Montagnier. Whatever his actual contribution, Montagnier got far more limelight than any of his colleagues following the isolation of the AIDS virus.[4]

Sabin wasted no time. In 1954 he wrote his first article about research on attenuated viruses. In 1956 he adminis-

tered his vaccine to roughly 9,000 monkeys, 150 chimpanzees, and 133 young adults in an Ohio prison. He enjoyed
the support of Merck, Sharp and Dohme, which gave him
some 25 million doses of each selected strain, something
for which, according to Vaughan, the company never received credit.

During a meeting in Stockholm to discuss polio vaccines in November 1955, Sabin presented results obtained
on a group of 80 volunteers, while Koprowski read a paper
detailing the findings of a trial enrolling 150 people.
Koprowski explained that in a group of children who had
been immunized previously, "antibodies remained for three
years following administration of a single dose."[5] He was
farther along than Cox or Sabin.

The various live, attenuated vaccines encountered two
obstacles, however. First, after Salk's injectable vaccine had
been proven effective, many people wondered if efforts to
develop another type of vaccine were justified. Sabin would
later tell the story of how his friend Tom Rivers, scientific
advisor to the National Foundation for Infantile Paralysis,
which had financed his research, advised him to dump his
strains in the sewer and abandon the project. Secondly, many
scientists and public health officials feared the attenuated
virus would revert to neurovirulence and cause cases of
polio. Their fears were not unfounded.

In 1956, George Dick, a microbiologist from Queens
University in Belfast, who had worked on the attenuated
yellow fever virus, suggested to Koprowski that they organize a field trial in Northern Ireland. The individuals who
received the vaccine suffered no undesirable side effects,
but virus in their stools produced paralysis in monkeys. Dick
voiced a warning about the risk that "by avoiding ten cases
of paralytic polio, we could later cause hundreds of cases of

paralysis," and recommended that Koprowski's vaccine not be used on a large scale.[6] His recommendations made the headlines.

In July 1957, the World Health Organization called a meeting of its Expert Committee on Polio, attended by Sabin and other researchers, to take stock of research on a live attenuated vaccine. The committee noted that trials to date had not caused undesirable side effects and recommended organizing large-scale trials, but under "extremely well-controlled conditions." It defined six criteria attenuated viral strains had to meet to guarantee they would be safe. The criteria had to be verified by several independent laboratories.

Koprowski adopted a line of reasoning that would no doubt be difficult to word today, when safety requirements are so much more stringent:

> Protection of man against a disease is obtained at a price; nothing in nature is given free, and all efforts should be made to reduce the cost of this payment. [...] The advocates of "safety" do not want to pay any price for immunization; yet, exactly, what are the costs one might have to pay for a method of immunization which would not only protect the vaccinated subject against the disease, but also may lead to elimination of poliomyelitis?[7]

Cox and Koprowski were so excited about the recommendation to organize large-scale field trials that they neglected the recommendation about the six criteria on attenuation, which would have prompted them to reexamine their strains. The work they had begun was already far along, so they continued it. Later some would note, with irony or bitterness, that Sabin did not run into any problems because his strains were in perfect compliance with the WHO criteria, which he had helped define.

In 1956, Koprowski had begun collaborations in the Belgian Congo, at the time a Belgian colony, with a Belgian virologist by the name of Ghislain Courtois. The two men had set up a facility to raise chimps to be used for research on hepatitis B and polio. In 1957, following the decisions of the WHO, Koprowski began a series of mass immunizations in Rwanda and the Congo. Nearly 250,000 people were vaccinated in the valley of the Ruzizi River; the researchers traveled up the river in dugout canoes, using a drum to call people to receive the vaccine. A polio epidemic that broke out in a village of 4,000 people was halted by immunizing all the villagers, which proved that the oral vaccine was effective in an emergency situation. The Belgian authorities then asked the scientists to immunize the children in Leopoldville and Stanleyville. Much ink would be spilled about these immunization campaigns forty years later, when a journalist attempted to link them to the AIDS epidemic.

From 1958 to 1960, Koprowski immunized 40,000 children in Germany and more than 7 million in Poland with attenuated type 1 or type 3 strains, or both (7.239 million with type 1 and 6.818 with type 3).

During the same period of time, Cox conducted trials in Florida and Berlin, Germany, that led to a high rate of paralysis due to vaccine-derived strains reverting to virulence, which prompted Lederle Labs to abandon all research with the strains Cox had used. In Germany, the father of a vaccinated child became infected with the vaccine-derived virus and died of polio.

In 1957, Sabin obtained a trivalent vaccine, that is, one containing attenuated strains of all three types of poliovirus. Over the next three years, he provided strains that were used to make vaccines against a single viral type (type 2 was administered to 200,000 children in Singapore in 1958) or against all three types. In the Soviet Union, a vaccine

OPV and HIV: A Hypothesis Disproved

For years rumors spread that HIV-1, the most wide-spread AIDS virus, had been transmitted from chim-panzees to humans during trials of an oral polio vaccine. This allegedly occurred during trials in the late 1950s conducted in the Congo by the Wistar Institute. In 1999, a British journalist wrote a book based on this hypothesis, claiming that the vaccines were contaminated when chimpanzee cells infected with the AIDS virus were used to grow the poliovirus. As a matter of fact, scientists have clearly established that HIV-1 comes from a Simian virus called SIV_{CPZ} found in chimpanzees, and HIV-2 comes from the virus called SIV_{SM} which infects mangabeys.

Several research laboratories have refuted the accusation. First, a team of American researchers demonstrated that all the current HIV-1 strains descend from a common ancestor, a strain dating back to 1930, that is, thirty years before the development of the OPV (*Science*, June 9, 2000). If these strains had evolved in chimpanzees before being transmitted to humans by vaccines, it would have been necessary for the cell cultures used to make the vaccine to be contaminated by nine different strains of the AIDS virus, which seems impossible. Scientists agree that HIV-1 passed from chimps to humans in the 1930s, and that since that time the virus has evolved in humans.

One year later, four articles showed that the poliovirus in the OPV doses used in the Congo by the Wistar Institute had been grown on cells from two species of macaques of Asian origin (*Nature*, April 26, 2001, and *Science*, April 27, 2001). Monkey cells, not chimpanzee

> **OPV and HIV (*continued*)**
>
> cells, were used, and the macaques captured in Asia do not become infected with SIV. Lastly, when old samples of the vaccine stored since the Congo trials were analyzed, no traces of HIV-1 or -2 were detected.

produced using strains provided by Sabin was administered to 15.2 million people in 1959 and 77.5 million in 1960, while 23 million people were vaccinated in several Eastern European countries. This marked a decisive step.

The speed and scope of the USSR's vaccine production were not unrelated to the cold war. In the mid-1950s, Anastas Mikoyan, a member of the Communist Party's Politburo, had thrown all his weight into organizing the fight against polio. The workers' and peasants' state could not appear do be doing less about the problem than the American capitalists.

Thomas Rivers tells the story of listening to a presentation by Professor Konstantine Vinokouroff of the Institute of Neurology of the Academy of Medical Sciences during the Second International Congress on Poliomyelitis, held in 1952 in Copenhagen:

> I will never forget him. He was a queer little fellow with a beard down to his upper chest. His talk was just as queer because he kept insisting that all the pioneer work in polio had first been done in Russia. That didn't bother anybody, but what was annoying was that he gave no indication that he was ever going to stop talking.[8]

Participants at the Congress were hardly convinced by Vinokouroff's claims that the Soviet Union had seen nothing like the dramatic epidemics that had struck in Western countries.

Sabin complained when his vaccine was at times referred to in the West as the "communist vaccine," but under the circumstances the vaccine was a guaranteed success, as if one of Stalin's Five-Year Plans were to exceed all expectations. The results of mass immunizations were published after being approved by the Presidium of the Academy of Medical Sciences. The Soviet researchers were pleased to announce them:

> In the Soviet Union there were no poliomyelitis cases on record which could be attributed to the immunization with live vaccine from the Sabin strains. [. . .] Specialists hold that under conditions of mass immunization there may be instances when vaccinations coincide with all kinds of symptoms produced by other affections. [. . .] The question of reactogenicity of the live vaccine appears to require some further detailed study, but it is not now of any great practical importance.[9]

More than 90 million people had been immunized; everyone was aware by then that the oral vaccine at times reverted to neurovirulence and caused cases of polio. In 1961, an exchange of letters between Sabin and Mikhail Chumakov, the leading scientist in charge of the Soviet program, bears witness to Sabin's irritation.

In 1968, Sabin once again had an opportunity to question his Soviet colleagues, when Boris Petrovsky, minister of health and member of the Russian Academy of Sciences and Academy of Medical Sciences, wrote in a history of public health in the USSR that two Soviet scientists, Mikhail Chumakov and Anatoli Smorodintsev, had developed the live attenuated polio vaccine. Sabin was furious; the president of the Academy of Medical Sciences explained to him that this was due to a mistake in the English translation of the book, which had been written in Russian.

Charles Mérieux, a leading French figure in the vaccine industry who followed developments concerning the polio vaccine very closely, was not entirely convinced. With his usual sense of wry observation, he wrote:

> When we asked the Soviet scientists to provide details and data, their only reply was that they had vaccinated 100 million people, and there were fewer and fewer cases of polio. They thought this was all we needed to know.[10]

When Albert Sabin asked Charles Mérieux to manufacture his vaccine on an industrial scale, Mérieux declined because he considered the results of the Russian experiment to be inadequate (although the Mérieux Institute would later produce the oral vaccine). But the massive utilization of the Sabin vaccine in communist countries established the vaccine internationally.

In 1958, the National Institutes of Health created a special committee on live polio vaccines, in charge of testing the strains authorized for the oral vaccine. The Koprowski and Cox strains were eliminated, as were those of Yale University, while the Sabin strains were selected for the three viral types. They rapidly became the only strains to be used worldwide.

Sabin had multiplied the number of passages in monkeys and in cell lines in order to improve the attenuation and stability of the viruses. The attenuated type 1 virus strain, for example, was derived from the Mahoney strain isolated in 1941. Salk made sixteen monkey kidney and monkey testicular passages, and other researchers had made fifteen or so more by 1953. Then in 1954 Sabin had the virus undergo another ten more passages followed by two further passes in 1956. Scientists at Merck, Sharp, and Dohme performed one additional passage on rhesus monkey kidney tissue culture before producing the vaccine.

Research to develop more stable strains continued, in particular for the type 3 attenuated virus, which reverted to neurovirulence more often than the other two.

In 1973–1974, a team of British scientists conducting research on monkeys observed that the type 3 strain used by Pfizer Laboratories, developed by virologist Robert Stones, presented less risk of reverting to a virulent strain than did the Sabin strain. In 1975, the Mérieux Institute, today sanofi-aventis, acquired all of Pfizer's biological material, including this type 3 attenuated strain, and distributed it to all the other vaccine manufacturers.

10

Revolution

in the

Production

of Vaccines

Lyon, France, 1955–1990

The production of polio vaccines marked a turning point in the vaccine industry. For the first time ever, huge quantities of a vaccine—tens of millions of doses—were in demand and manufacturers needed to be both imaginative and daring to meet this challenge.

The story of the industrial development of any product is rarely a public affair. Such episodes in the history of medicine are rarely written down, perhaps to protect industrial secrets, out of habit, or simply because no one looks into them.

We had the good fortune of meeting and interviewing former scientists, technicians, directors, and employees of the Connaught Laboratories in Canada and the Mérieux Institute in France. Today these two companies are both part of sanofi-aventis, the world's largest private manufacturer of oral and injectable polio vaccines. They both played a critical role in the history of the polio vaccine. As was explained in previous chapters, Connaught supplied the viral fluids that made the Francis Field Trial of the Salk vaccine possible, while the Mérieux Institute moved vaccine production to the industrial scale.

Shortly before his death on January 19, 2001, we spoke to Dr. Charles Mérieux, who led the Mérieux Institute as it took its first steps into the world of human vaccines. He told us the story of this "extraordinary adventure."

During one of his many journeys across the Atlantic, in 1955 Charles Mérieux met Jonas Salk, Albert Sabin, and Hilary Koprowski. He was struck by the fact that the biologists of the world did not speak a common language. How, then, could they possibly establish international standards to guarantee basic safety for candidate vaccines? "With no common standards to establish and test vaccines and sera," said Charles Mérieux, "scientists were unable to evaluate or compare them, which meant they could not import or export them. As a result, it was impossible to develop international cooperation or define a coherent policy for worldwide prevention."[1]

Dr. Mérieux wanted to organize a congress on biological standards, which he succeeded in doing in 1956, in the Lyon city hall, thanks to the support of Édouard Herriot, the then-prime minister of France and former mayor of the city of Lyon. In the thick of the cold war, the presence of American scientists gave the encounter an international flavor.

After the congress, in 1957, Charles Mérieux became interested in an injectable vaccine developed by Pierre Lépine, a scientist at the Pasteur Institute. Lépine had developed a vaccine that, although based on the same inactivation principle as Salk's IPV, was not the same vaccine. The virus in the vaccine was inactivated twice.

Bernard Montagnon, former head of viral production at the Mérieux Institute, explained: "In addition to formalin, the Lépine vaccine used betapropiolactone, which speeded up the inactivation process. It took just four days to inactivate the Lépine vaccine, compared to twelve for the Salk vaccine. The chemical agent betapropiolactone had another advantage: it killed the viruses that were likely to contaminate the monkey kidney cells."

This was not the case when formalin was used alone. The Merck, Sharp, and Dohme Laboratories were forced to abandon attempts to produce a killed vaccine when, in 1960, they discovered that a simian virus, SV 40, was not destroyed by formalin and contaminated simian cell cultures.

In twenty years, Lépine produced several million doses of vaccine for the Pasteur Institute at Marnes-la-Coquette. Convinced that the vaccine was totally safe, Charles Mérieux decided to begin production. The polio vaccine was the first human vaccine to be produced by the Mérieux Institute.

The first cell cultures used to make the French IPV vaccine came from dog-faced (cynocephalus) baboons; subsequently patas and vervet monkey cells were used. The type 1 virus was made with a viral strain isolated in the sewage water of Paris. The steps after isolation—inactivation and controls of the vaccine—were very similar to the methods the Mérieux Institute had developed to manufacture a veterinary vaccine to prevent foot-and-mouth disease.

Every day at six A.M., the laboratory technicians arrived at the animal facility to remove monkey kidneys. Wearing sterile gowns, they put the kidneys in Petri dishes, which were then transported in ice chests. Bernard Fanget, one of the technicians in the early days, described how they "trypsinized" the monkey kidneys. "After cutting them into small pieces and mincing the tissue, we used an enzyme called trypsin, which separated the cells and enabled us to obtain a cellular suspension."

The suspension was then poured into stainless steel tanks containing growth medium with all the necessary nutrients for cell proliferation: proteins, vitamins, amino acids, salt, sugars, and so on. Next, the technicians transferred the suspension into Roux dishes to obtain a stationary cell culture. The Roux dishes were placed horizontally on a cart and transported into rooms where the temperature was maintained at 37°C (98.6°F). After a few days, a layer of cells formed. The technicians removed the growth medium in which cell multiplication had taken place and replaced it with fresh medium. They introduced the poliovirus, which multiplied 10,000 times.

"The last step of the operation consisted of purifying the fluids by removing the cellular debris to obtain a suspension containing billions of viral particles," explained Bernard Fanget.

Purification is a critical step. This is also true for viral inactivation, as is attested to by the difficulties experienced by John Beale at Glaxo in 1956. Active polio virus was found in 7.5 percent of vaccine lots after inactivation, following two to three weeks of culture. Scientists at the company realized that the problem had begun when the glassworker who made their special filters had left the company. Clumps of cellular debris were preventing the virus from being inactivated.

It took about one week to bring the cell culture to the right level and produce the viral suspension for each type of virus (types 1, 2, and 3). Before blending the three serotypes to produce a trivalent vaccine, each monovalent batch was tested for safety and immunogenicity, meaning that it induced the production of antibodies. Other tests were performed on the trivalent preparation, which increased the time required to produce the vaccine. More than one hundred days went by between the time the monkeys were sacrificed and the moment the vaccine was filled into ampuls. A final control was performed on a sample from each lot.

In the 1960s, the laboratory that manufactured the Lépine vaccine in Marcy l'Etoile, in the suburbs of Lyon, employed some thirty people who produced nearly five million doses of vaccine per year.

"For twenty-five years, we sacrificed the equivalent of 20,000 monkeys to produce the polio vaccine," said Charles Mérieux. "To obtain the greatest good from the sacrifice of the monkeys, we set up a collaboration with medical research organizations in Lyon. We loaned them the monkeys, which their scientists used to attempt the first organ transplants. This allowed them to perfect their techniques before applying them to humans and is one of the reasons the surgeons in Lyon soon acquired a solid reputation in the field of organ transplants. They were pioneers in kidney, liver, and heart transplants."

In 1960 a decree was issued making polio vaccination mandatory in France. Thanks to DT Polio, a combination vaccine that protected against polio, diphtheria, and tetanus, the Mérieux Institute soon earned a name for itself in France in the field of pediatric vaccination. At the time, it was impossible to create a single vaccine containing the four required childhood vaccines—diphtheria, tetanus, polio, and whooping cough (pertussis)—due to a problem of preservative incompatibility.

Michel Galy, former general manager of the Mérieux Institute, recalled: "I was on a journey to the United States with Charles Mérieux. We had come to visit the Lederle Laboratories. We were deep in discussion with the director of the company when Charles Mérieux interrupted the conversation, pointing to a syringe on the desk."

It was a dual-chamber syringe containing two different products stored separately inside the syringe but injected in a single shot. Charles Mérieux had a vision: He imagined the DTP coq vaccine (diphtheria, tetanus, pertussis) on one side and the polio vaccine on the other. In 1964, the Mérieux Institute marketed this combination in a dual-chamber syringe.

In the early 1960s the Mérieux Institute began to produce the oral polio vaccine (OPV) developed by Albert Sabin. At that point, Charles Mérieux considered the OPV had proven itself.

"Since my company was private and independent, I was free to use my own judgment and make my own choices," said Charles Mérieux. "I knew that the evidence in favor of the Sabin vaccine was continuing to accumulate. So much so that finally I decided that we, too, should manufacture the OPV. Albert Sabin of course accepted, since he had initially approached us with this idea. I invited him and all the European specialists to Lyon. During their encounter, many presentations confirmed that Sabin's vaccine was safe and that it would be very complex to standardize it."

The poliovirus was cultured on monkey kidney cells for the oral polio vaccine, just as for the IPV. The oral vaccine is theoretically easier to make because it does not require the inactivation phase. Instead, a viral suspension produced by culturing attenuated (weakened) strains of the virus is diluted to obtain the right concentration.

Lot controls were the main challenge for OPV production. Control operations had to be stepped up to produce vaccines on an industrial scale; it was at this time that controls took on such importance for the medical and pharmaceutical industries.

"Gradually, the new vaccine gained ground and was used in mass immunization campaigns, although France, the Netherlands, and the Scandinavian countries remained faithful to the injectable vaccine," said Charles Mérieux. "In addition, as I expected from the outset, rather than competing, the two formulations—Lépine and Sabin—turned out to be complementary. Often doctors would give the first vaccination by injection, and then follow up with oral boosters, which were easier to administer."

Jonas Salk, still troubled by the Cutter incident, was eager to reestablish his inactivated vaccine, especially in the United States. At the World Health Organization, Frank Perkins advised him to meet Charles Mérieux, who might be able to help him industrialize the vaccine.

Said Charles Mérieux: "Jonas Salk knew that his vaccine would make a comeback, but the commercial laboratories had all abandoned him. Thanks to Tetracoq, we were the only company to produce the injectable polio vaccine on an industrial scale, while maintaining production of the oral vaccine."

Jonas Salk collaborated with Dutch researchers from the RIVM, the National Institute of Public Health and the Environment, where an engineer by the name of Toon Van Wezel had developed a technique to grow cells on "microcarriers," micro-beads which are floating, suspended in the growth medium. This invention greatly increased the number of cells that could be grown in a given volume.

Adherent cells (such as those used to make the polio vaccine) attach to a solid surface and multiply. Regardless of the volume it holds, if the base of a flask measures 10 cm × 10 cm, the flask will be able to contain no more than 100 cm^2 of cells. When, instead, the cells are grown on the spherical surface of microcarriers suspended in a liquid, the total available surface is enormous, and yet the flask takes up little space and requires only a limited amount of growth medium, which is very expensive. In the mind of Charles Mérieux, Van Wezel's discovery represented "a new revolution, whose repercussions were comparable to those of Frenckel's discovery," that the virus of foot-and-mouth disease could be grown in cultures made from cow tongue epithelial cells.

Once this technique had been adapted to the production of polio vaccines, it revolutionized the production of all other vaccines.

The Mérieux Institute had no choice but to build its own equipment at the production site. "We took a shot in the dark," said Michel Galy. The team developed all the equipment needed for vaccine production, and later made it fully automated.

Jonas Salk and Charles Mérieux and his team were in the midst of preparing an important breakthrough: a system to manufacture IPV without using live animals. Vaccine production had been considerably limited by the need to culture monkey kidney cells. "A new vaccine that would be produced from a cell that we could build up stocks of. Ultimately, this would mean we did not have to sacrifice any animals. It was clearly the solution for the future," said Charles Mérieux.

Salk wanted to use continuous cell lines. These cell lines came from "transformed" green monkey cells and could reproduce for an extended period of time *in vitro*, whereas normal cells will divide only a limited number of times. Normal cells die after a few generations, meaning the culture process must be started all over again. By comparison, cells in continuous cell lines continue to multiply and the cell lines can be divided as often as necessary.

Using such cell lines to manufacture human vaccines would, however, require convincing the scientific community of their safety. It feared that this practice might entail unacceptable risks because cells from the lines that could pass into the vaccine could potentially become carcinogenic in vaccinated individuals.

In 1977, Jonas Salk and Philippe Stoeckel, the head of the Association for the Promotion of Preventive Medicine— created by Jacques Monod and Charles Mérieux in 1972— visited Paul Albrecht's laboratory at the National Institutes of Health in Bethesda, Maryland. They identified three candidate cell lines: Vero, LLCMK2, and CV1; they evaluated each of these for its nontumorigenic character. They determined the nutrients required for their development, with a view to using the cell lines for industrial production. They finally chose the Vero cell line.[2]

A new injectable polio vaccine (IPV) formula was developed at the National Institute of Public Health and the Environment (RIVM) in the Netherlands by Toon Van Wezel, under the direction of Hans Cohen. The virus was concentrated and purified and combined with formalin; its antigenic content was then calibrated for the three serological types. The "enhanced" vaccine, as it was called, was more economical and reduced the risk of error during inactivation.

At about the same time, Jonas Salk, Hans Cohen, and Charles Mérieux founded the Forum for the Advancement of Immunization Research, or FAIR, with the aim of standardizing vaccines.

The forum coordinated clinical trials of the enhanced IPV vaccine. Its founders wanted to determine the minimum doses of each of the three viral types required to obtain protective immunity for anyone who received the vaccine. The findings were presented by the trial coordinators at a symposium held in late August 1981 and were published in 1982. They showed that 40 units of type 1, 8 units of type 2, and 32 units of type 3 were sufficient to induce immunity among all vaccinated individuals. The 40–8–32 ratio became the standard for all polio vaccines produced worldwide.

With Paul Albrecht, the forum also coordinated a study for the standardization of seroneutralization techniques used in the laboratory to determine the immunity induced by the vaccine. Some thirty laboratories took part in this study.

To ensure that IPV vaccines were identical throughout the world, as well as to guarantee their safety, it was also essential to define standards for cell culturing. At a meeting in 1984, organized by John Petricciani of the NIH, two essential criteria were adopted. From then on, all vaccine manufacturers had to respect these criteria to ensure the complete safety of vaccines produced on cell lines:

- the quantity of residual cellular DNA must be less than 100 pg per dose of vaccine, which corresponds to the genome of one cell
- the various purification phases must reduce the quantity of cellular DNA by a factor of 10^{-8}, from the fluids in the tanks to the final product.

First microcarriers, now Vero cells: a revolution at the Mérieux Institute! Shelves upon shelves of Roux dishes, which required tedious, time-consuming handling, were traded for stainless steel tanks filled with microcarriers. Inside the tanks, Vero cells replaced monkey kidney cells. The new techniques brought an end to the days of capturing monkeys in the savannahs and forests of Africa. The mass production of polio vaccines was underway. By 1987, the institute's annual production of IPV on Vero cells had reached nearly 25 million doses.

Bernard Montagnon summarized the lessons of this period in the company's history: "In six years, the Mérieux

Institute had met the objective set by Jonas Salk: the regional eradication of the poliovirus using IPV."

Very quickly, OPV was also produced on Vero cells and the WHO and UNICEF asked the Mérieux Institute to produce large quantities of vaccine, with all the necessary guarantees of safety. "The WHO experts were afraid our processes would lead to a selection of virulent viral particles," recalled Bernard Montagnon. "They asked us to show them proof, on 300,000 subjects, that the pharmacovigilance of the attenuated vaccine was satisfactory. And we did." UNICEF began using the vaccine in developing countries in August 1989 for the polio eradication campaign.

With regulatory demands becoming stricter by the day, the production of vaccines is an increasingly difficult business. Vaccines are made with biological products, using living materials and, for this reason, will always be subject to a certain degree of variability and unpredictability. Production facilities have been completely rebuilt to meet draconian safety standards. While for a drug, the health authorities must approve the active ingredient and the production sites, each batch of vaccine must be authorized for release by the authorities and facilities are inspected in great detail on a regular basis.

Today an average of five years goes by from the moment a company decides to invest in a production facility and when it sells its first dose of vaccine. The production cycle for a vaccine varies from one to two years, and 70 percent of this time is devoted to controls. The vaccine industry is therefore highly capitalistic, for products whose selling price is generally not high.

Vaccines are, moreover, administered to individuals in good health. Society's threshold of tolerance for side effects is much lower than for drugs given to treat a disease that may be painful or debilitating, and even more so if the disease is deadly. The industrial risk of producing a vaccine has grown considerably as health safety standards have become increasingly strict.

Given the pressure due to these three factors—regulatory standards, capital investment, and industrial risk—the number of vaccine producers has dwindled, either because companies go out of business, are absorbed in a merger, or decide to focus their activities on the purely pharmaceutical sector. Although most patents fell into the public domain years ago, there are no generic vaccines. The vaccine industry is probably the only industrial sector where demand is consistently greater than supply. The WHO keeps a list of twenty or so vaccine producers approved to sell to United Nation organizations, but in reality four major private vaccine producers dominate the world market: sanofi-aventis, Merck, Wyeth, and GlaxoSmithKline.

The number of manufacturers who make the polio vaccine has followed this general trend. In the United States, for the first few decades of OPV production, Merck, Wyeth, Pfizer, and Lederle marketed the vaccine. Today only Wyeth, which absorbed Lederle, continues to produce OPV. Five companies in the United States and one in Canada produced IPV; today sanofi-aventis is the only company that continues to market IPV for all of North America.

11

Polio

Programmed for Defeat

India, January 2001

Aligarh, Uttar Pradesh, Sunday, January 21, 2001, 7:30 A.M. In the courtyard of the local branch office of the Ministry of Health of Uttar Pradesh, Archana Mudger is standing next to a yellow school bus on loan for the day, giving out orders. The nineteen-year-old history student is surrounded by a crowd of mothers and mostly male students who tower above her, yet she is in her element. All eyes are on her; everyone listens intently, slightly anxious. The young woman holds a folder from which she draws out detailed, hand-drawn maps of some of Aligarh's neighborhoods—not places people are usually keen to venture into.

Archana and her team are wearing caps emblazoned with the motto "Kick polio out of India" written in Hindi letters. Inside the bus are ice chests piled one on top of another. They are equipped with shoulder straps and display the campaign logo, "Pulse Polio," the name given in India to the Global Polio Eradication Initiative launched by the World Health Organization in 1988. Inside the containers are vials of OPV, the oral vaccine used for the immunization campaigns that seek to rid the planet of the poliomyelitis virus.

Archana chairs a local organization called Shivam Gramy Smatrari, whose most active members are surrounding her this morning. "My brother founded the organization a year and a half ago to help those whom no one else takes care of," says the young woman. "Then he died and I took over. We have about three hundred members, mainly students, but also some mothers and housewives. They're all from Aligarh's middle classes. The government distributes vaccines against polio, but they mainly benefit the more fortunate classes. We want to reach the neediest."

Kamal Singhal is a surveillance medical officer (SMO). As the physician in charge of the polio eradication campaign in the Aligarh region, he explains that cases of polio occur most often in the poorest neighborhoods, where population density is high. The virus also circulates in better-off areas, but since hygiene is better and immunization rates are higher, few people there contract the disease.

"In Aligarh," says Dr. Singhal, "the health services employ very few people, so we need nongovernmental organizations for the vaccination campaigns. In the urban areas there are eighteen public health workers for every one million inhabitants, and an average of twenty for every one million inhabitants in the countryside.

"On the first National Immunization Day [NID] in which the Shivam organization participated, they manned fifteen vaccination booths. They did an excellent job. All the volunteers know what to do. The maps of the areas they had to cover were extremely detailed. For the next Immunization Days, we allotted them forty-three vaccination booths. The Shivam workers are young, energetic, and enthusiastic and we've assigned them to the toughest neighborhoods."

On this January morning, the well-dressed, well-fed Hindu students of Shivam set out for Maqdum Najr, a predominantly Muslim neighborhood. In India, half of all polio cases affect Muslims even though Muslims represent only 10 to 15 percent of the population. They are the country's poorest minority. In the community that the Shivam volunteers will be combing, nearly 100 percent of the population is illiterate, almost no one has running water, and there is no sewage system. Shanties with corrugated iron roofs, where people freeze in winter and swelter in summer, crowd the sides of potholed roads, dotted with pools of murky water.

The yellow bus drops off the volunteers at the vaccination sites, where other members of the organization meet them. They roll out banners with "National Polio Immunization Day" written in Hindi and hang up posters that proclaim, "Our only aim: free Aligarh of polio" in Hindi and in Urdu, the language spoken by the Muslim community. They set up folding tables where they stack sheets of paper on which they will keep a record of the children they immunize. Then they remove a few vials of vaccine from one of the ice chests.

The waiting crowd makes a rush for the booth. Mothers carry their babies forward. Children who are big enough to walk elbow their way to the front. A student squeezes three drops into the first open mouth, then into another, and another. A second student colors one finger on every vaccinated child with a streak of blue paint so that the same child does not receive more than one dose. It is impossible to count the number of little mouths that receive the three cherry-flavored drops. The statistics will be inexact, but what counts is to vaccinate as many children as possible.

The vaccinators in Aligarh are at the end of a long chain: John Enders, the March of Dimes volunteers, Jonas Salk, and Albert Sabin; the employees working in the factories of vaccine producers; epidemiologists, doctors, and volunteers—all joined together in a chain of tens of thousands of individuals stretching over half a century, culminating in this scene of merry chaos to protect the poorest of children from the suffering caused by polio.

In India, a National Immunization Day mobilizes 2.7 million volunteers, who immunize 140 million children at 650,000 sites. In Aligarh, besides the Sivam Organization, the members of Gaia Tri Pariwan, a branch of the Hindu religion, and the students of the Islamic School of Medicine also join in.

In 2000, 550 million children were vaccinated during the National Immunization Days organized by local authorities in eighty-two countries, with the help of the WHO and the other partners in the eradication campaign. The National Immunization Days are a vital aspect of the Global Polio Eradication Initiative launched in Geneva on May 13, 1988, by the WHO during a historic General Assembly.

The World Health Organization's decision was a continuation of the Expanded Program on Immunization, which aimed to vaccinate as many children as possible, throughout the world, against the main vaccine-preventable diseases: measles, diphtheria, whooping cough (pertussis), tetanus, tuberculosis, and polio. The WHO initiative followed the "PolioPlus" campaign launched by Rotary International in 1985.

William Sergeant, chairman of Rotary International's PolioPlus Committee, explains what led the organization to join the struggle against polio. "Until 1978, Rotary clubs acted individually in their communities. Then we decided to do something that would involve all members worldwide, something important that clubs couldn't do alone. The eradication of a disease corresponded to our will to do something together, and gradually we reached the conclusion that the disease should be polio. Our choice had a great deal to do with the fact that polio affects little people, the most innocent members of society. We still had Rotary leaders who remembered the terribly crippling effects of polio in the U.S.

"When we launched the program in 1985, we estimated that if we raised $120 million, we would buy vaccines for developing countries over five years. This sounded impossible to some Rotarians. The first surprise was that we raised $247 million, which was incredible!

"This caused us to change our entire outlook. We couldn't just go out and buy $247 million worth of vaccines and distribute them. We had a long haul ahead of us. Not only the fight against polio, but perhaps its eradication, was on the agenda. We invested this money, and decided to continue with fund-raising. Rotary's support, and our success, were crucial for the resolution adopted by the WHO in 1988."

By June 30, 2000, Rotary had donated a total of $378 million to the fight against polio in 122 countries. The organization is committed to raising $500 million all together by 2005. Over one million Rotary members worldwide have been directly involved in the polio eradication campaign.

"I don't think we realized just how much we would have to do, nor did we understand the obstacles we had to overcome," says William Sergeant. "We didn't know what we would have to do besides coming up with money to buy vaccine. As a matter of fact, today most of our expenditure is not on vaccines, but on surveillance activities, cold chain support, and social mobilization. And Rotarians participate in National Immunization Days."

Members of Rotary are mostly business and professional men and women, politicians, teachers, and other commu-

---

A Brief History of Rotary

Rotary was founded on February 23, 1905, in Chicago by Paul P. Harris, an attorney who wanted to recapture in a professional club some of the friendly spirit he had grown up with in the small towns of his youth. The club was named "Rotary" because members rotated meetings among their various places of business.

Rotary rapidly became very popular. By 1921 Rotary clubs had been created on six continents. According to Rotary International, a conference it organized in London in 1942 planted the seeds for the development of UNESCO after World War II.

Today, 1.2 million Rotarians belong to some 29,000 clubs in over 160 countries. The Rotary Foundation's annual budget of approximately $80 million is used to support humanitarian and educational programs and to provide grants.

---

nity leaders in industrialized countries. Their influence contributes to the advancement of the Global Polio Eradication Initiative.

"Rotary also takes steps to convince the leaders of polio-free countries that it is in their best interest to eradicate polio, and to urge them to provide money," explains William Sergeant. "Rotary members were among those who encouraged the U.S. Congress to increase its aid. In 1995, Congress had allocated $11 million for polio eradication. The current contribution is $112 million."

Another key partner in the Global Polio Eradication Campaign, the Centers for Disease Control and Prevention, was also involved in polio eradication prior to 1988.

Says Dr. Steve Cochi of the CDC: "We began working

on the polio initiative in the Americas by participating in the campaign launched by the Pan American Health Organization in 1985. The western hemisphere was the testing ground for the key strategies for polio eradication. We provide technical support for the Initiative. Our reference laboratory supports the worldwide network of 147 laboratories accredited by the WHO for polio surveillance. This is the largest network of laboratories ever established. Some of our specialists are on loan to the WHO and UNICEF. We work in close partnership with the core partners, the WHO, Rotary, and UNICEF."

The certified eradication of smallpox, declared by the Thirty-third World Health Assembly on May 8, 1980, is the precedent most often cited in the effort to rally support for the fight against polio. Nearly forty years after launch of the campaign to eradicate smallpox in the 1960s, many people have forgotten some of the difficulties this program encountered.

This successful eradication program was preceded by several failed attempts to eliminate other diseases. In 1909, the Rockefeller Sanitary Commission launched a campaign to eradicate hookworm, a parasite that causes anemia. In the 1950s, campaigns were mounted to eradicate yaws (a tropical disease caused by a bacterium similar to that which causes syphilis) and malaria; these efforts were abandoned in 1970. A new form of injectable, long-acting, single-dose penicillin raised hopes of eliminating yaws. Officials thought malaria could be eradicated by eliminating the vector, the Anopheles mosquito, through DDT spraying. For fifteen years, the WHO allocated five hundred people and over one-third of its expenditures to the malaria eradication program—in vain. Efforts to eradicate yellow fever were also abandoned in the late 1970s when scientists realized the virus survived in insects.

After so many disappointments, it was an uphill battle to garner the support necessary for the eradication of smallpox. Donald A. Henderson, a professor at Johns Hopkins University in Baltimore, Maryland, and founding director, Center for Civilian Biodefense Strategies, who led the smallpox eradication campaign, explains:

> A number of endemic countries were themselves persuaded only with difficulty to participate in the program; the industrialized countries were reluctant contributors and UNICEF, so helpful to the prior malaria program, decided that it wanted nothing to do with another eradication program and stated that it would make no contributions. Several countries did make donations of vaccine and the West African program, directed by the U.S. Communicable Disease Center, was a critical addition. However, cash donations to the WHO during the first seven years of the smallpox program, 1967–73, amounted to exactly $79,500.

The author adds:

> Eradication was achieved by only the narrowest of margins. Its progress in many parts of the world and at different times wavered between success and disaster, often only to be decided by quixotic circumstance or extraordinary performances by field staff.[1]

To eliminate an infectious disease from the surface of the planet, a number of conditions must be met. Smallpox fit all the criteria: first, there was no animal reservoir for the virus (by contrast, today it would be impossible to eradicate yellow fever or influenza because the virus that infects humans also affects animals that cannot be vaccinated); second, smallpox epidemics were easy to monitor since the symptoms of the disease never go unnoticed; and finally,

Closer to Dracunculiasis Eradication

Dracunculiasis, which is prevalent in rural areas, is caused by the Guinea worm or the Medina filiary, a parasitic Nematode, which infects humans through drinking water.

The worm grows for about one year inside the body of an infected person, reaching a length of 60 to 90 cm before emerging through the skin. The female worm deposits immature larvae in water, where they are eaten by small crustaceans, in which the larvae undergo two molts. Humans are infected when they drink water containing these invertebrates. There is no treatment for the disease.

The Dracunculiasis Eradication Program, launched in 1980, set out to provide clean drinking water to populations at risk and to teach people to filter or boil their water.

Between 1986 and 1997, the incidence of dracunculiasis dropped by 97 percent, going from an estimated 3.2 million cases to fewer than 100,000. The parasite has been wiped out in India and Pakistan. It is still present in less than 10,000 villages, over half of which are in Sudan, where civil war blocks prevention campaigns. Most of the remaining cases are found in Burkina Faso, Ghana, Niger, and Nigeria.

According to D. R. Hopkins of the Carter Center in Atlanta, in addition to slowing the incidence of the disease, "The program has already produced many indirect benefits such as improved agricultural production and school attendance, extensive provision of clean drinking water, mobilization of endemic communities, and improved care of infants."

Source: "Perspectives from the Dracunculiasis Eradication Programme," *MMWR* 48, Suppl. (December 31, 1999), CDC.

the vaccine was effective enough to stop the transmission of the virus.

Poliomyelitis meets these criteria, but it also involves thornier problems, as Dr. Steve Cochi of the CDC explains:

> One of the major differences is that when the smallpox eradication program began, most of the world was already smallpox-free. There were only about 30 countries that still had smallpox, in contrast to the 125 countries that had polio when we began the Polio Initiative. The challenge of the Polio Initiative is magnified by the fact that the poliovirus spreads silently. The number of carriers is far higher than the number of paralytic cases of polio, making it much harder to track the spread of an epidemic. With smallpox, the characteristic skin rash of infected individuals made them easily recognizable. Multiple doses of polio vaccine are required to protect against the disease, whereas for smallpox a single dose sufficed.

All those involved in overseeing the Global Polio Eradication Initiative will readily point out that what gives the initiative its best chance of success is the tremendous mobilization on which it is based. The struggle to fight polio has combined people's enthusiastic response to the March of Dimes and the Francis Field Trial of the Salk vaccine with the logistic capabilities of governments and international organizations. Alongside the WHO, which acts as the umbrella organization, Rotary, without whose financial and human support nothing would be possible, and the CDC, which provide their expertise, the United Nations Children's Fund (UNICEF, formerly United Nations International Children's Emergency Fund) is the fourth major partner in the campaign.

Carol Bellamy, executive director of UNICEF, explains

the role her organization plays: "UNICEF purchases the vaccines and ensures the cold chain will be maintained. We also provide training for health workers involved in immunization and contribute to awareness-raising campaigns."
Much of the stock of vaccines purchased by UNICEF is stored in its warehouses in Amsterdam, until it is dispatched to the sites where it is needed. As is true of all the vaccines included in the Expanded Program on Immunization (EPI), UNICEF negotiates with vaccine producers to obtain the best possible conditions in terms of price and quantities.

The polio eradication strategy is based, above all, on the routine vaccination of young children. In many industrialized countries, the polio vaccine is one of the vaccines that is either mandatory or recommended. Polio vaccination is included in the immunization programs implemented in developing countries by UNICEF and the WHO, within the framework of the Expanded Program on Immunization.

In 1988, it was estimated that 60 percent of all children worldwide were completely immunized, by their first birthday, against polio, diphtheria, pertussis, tetanus, measles, and tuberculosis. This is ten times the figure for 1974, when the EPI was launched. Such spectacular progress was one of the arguments put forward to support the launch of the Polio Eradication Initiative.

In 1999, polio immunization coverage—the estimated percentage of children under one year of age who have received all the necessary doses of polio vaccine—was over 78 percent. However, coverage varied greatly according to geographical location: 11 percent in Afghanistan, 12 percent in Guinea-Bissau, and around 20 percent in five other African countries, 90 percent in the United States and over 95 percent in most industrialized countries. Immunization coverage by age two reached 97.2 percent in France in 1998. The WHO targets an immunization coverage of 90 percent

Table 11.1
Use of IPV and OPV Worldwide

	Number of Countries	Annual Births (in millions)
IPV alone	22	6.8
IPV and OPV	8	0.5
Expected to shift		
soon from OPV to IPV	4	1.8
OPV alone	178	122.7

Source: World Health Organization, 2002.

worldwide for all the vaccines in the EPI, including polio. Specialists estimate that coverage of at least 85 percent is necessary to prevent the virus from circulating.

Depending on the country, routine immunization uses the oral vaccine developed by Albert Sabin (OPV), the injectable vaccine based on Jonas Salk's method (IPV), or a combination of the two. Virtually all developing countries use OPV, for example, while in France the oral vaccine would be used only in the event of an epidemic, with the injectable vaccine recommended for mandatory vaccination. With the global progress toward polio eradication, all Canadian provinces recently changed from routine OPV immunization to IPV. Similarly, until recently, the recommendations of U.S. authorities varied: OPV alone, IPV alone, or two doses of IPV followed by two doses of OPV. Since January 2000, the use of the injectable vaccine is recommended for all four doses in the immunization schedule, again because of the progress toward global eradication.

The main argument for using IPV rather than OPV is that with IPV there is no risk of vaccine-associated polio as the attenuated strain used for OPV can rarely revert to virulence and cause poliomyelitic paralysis. Between 1980 and 1994, on average, eight cases of vaccine-associated poliomyelitis were recorded annually in the United States. The number of cases of the disease associated with the vaccine is estimated at one for every 750,000 children who receive their first dose.

Organizing National Immunization Days, like the campaign in the streets of Aligarh in which Archana and her friends participated, is the second part of the Global Polio Eradication Initiative strategy. The operation is repeated several times a year to simultaneously boost population immunity while increasing the likelihood that every child will get the four doses required for effective and lasting immunization. The vaccinators immunize all children under five years of age that they meet, regardless of the number of doses they have already received.

Unfortunately, not all mothers are able to bring their children to the vaccination booths. Perhaps they are unaware of the Immunization Day or they do not understand how important vaccination is, or perhaps they fear the vaccines. The third element in the WHO's strategy is therefore referred to as "mop-up campaigns."

On January 22, the members of Shivam and of Gaia Tripavar and the students of the Islamic School of Medicine of Aligarh knocked on all the doors of the town, went into all the shanties, and explored every nook and cranny of the neighborhoods to which they had been assigned. Hundreds of thousands of volunteers did the same throughout the country.

They asked, "How many children under five live here?" and jotted down the reply in a notebook. "Can you bring them to us?" they continued. One of the volunteers squeezed three drops of the vaccine into the mouth of each child. Another completed the record in the notebook and made chalk marks on the door or wall of the home, to show how many children had been immunized.

Such immunization campaigns make use of the OPV. Bruce Aylward, the WHO international coordinator for the Global Polio Eradication Initiative, explains the benefits of OPV compared to IPV:

The two vaccines confer different types of immunity. OPV helps to produce antibodies in the intestine, which is very useful because that is how children become infected. So the antibodies are right at the site of the infection. The injectable vaccine provides what we call humoral immunity, i.e., antibodies that circulate in the blood and are not always as effective as antibodies in the intestines when it comes to stopping a polio outbreak. This characteristic of the OPV has made it essential to the global eradication initiative.

The second major difference is in the logistics of the delivery. The OPV can be given by virtually anyone, after a few minutes of simple instruction. This makes it easy to conduct these massive campaigns around the world—campaigns which included ten million volunteer vaccinators in the year 2001 alone. The IPV requires a needle and syringe, and one has to be very careful to ensure that vaccination with this method is safe.

The third difference lies in the cost. The OPV is the only vaccine used in developing countries, and the only one purchased by UNICEF. Therefore there is a special negotiated price. In contrast, IPV is substantially more expensive, in part because no price has been negotiated for use in the developing country setting.

Because OPV uses an attenuated, living virus, it has another crucial advantage: it can reach children who slip through the nets of the immunization campaigns. The vaccine virus multiplies in the digestive tract and leaves the body through the stools, infecting people who live around the vaccinated children. This chain of events means that "escapees" are vaccinated indirectly.

"The oral vaccine provides contact immunization," explains Pierre Morgon, former vice president of marketing, sanofi-aventis International. "After the initial dose, the vaccine protects the intestinal tissues, and encourages the multiplication of the viral strain, which leaves the body via the stools and can be transmitted to others. Children who have gone off to look after the goats in the mountains can acquire the vaccine-derived strains from their playmates when they return to their village. Starting with a single vaccinated child, we can hope that others will be immunized as well."

Poor hygiene actually increases indirect immunization. The worse the conditions of hygiene, the greater the chances of this type of exposure.

———

The Global Polio Eradication Initiative has achieved staggering results. The estimated number of polio cases diminished by 99 percent between 1988 and 2000, dropping from 350,000 to 3,500 annually. In 1988, the wild poliovirus was circulating in 125 countries: all the African countries, nearly all the Asian countries, most of Central and South America, the Soviet Union, France, and Spain. By the end of 2002, it had been limited to 7 countries.

In 1991, a three-year-old Peruvian boy, Luis Fermin Tenorio, was the last child paralyzed by wild poliomyelitis virus in the Americas, which were certified polio-free in 1994. In March 1997, a fifteen-month-old Cambodian girl, Mum Chanty, was the last victim in the WHO Western Pacific Region, certified polio-free in October 2000. The next region expected to be considered polio-free is Europe, where it appears that the last case of paralysis due to a nonimported wild virus was contracted by a young Turkish boy, Melik Minas, who fell ill in November 1998 when he was two and a half years old.

On March 30, 2001, the *Morbidity and Mortality Weekly Report*, the CDC newsletter, announced that the poliovirus type 2 had disappeared. The last countries where this type of virus was identified by analyzing the stools of affected individuals were Afghanistan and Pakistan in 1997, Nigeria in 1998, and India in 1999. The last reported case of a wild virus type 2 occurred in the Indian state of Bihar in October 1999.

Before the advent of polio vaccination, the wild virus type 2, like the other two types, was to be found throughout the world. The CDC attributes its rapid diminution and disappearance to the high immunogenicity of the type 2 strain of the oral vaccine—its efficacy as a vaccine—and to the efficient spread of the vaccine-derived strain, which ensures the spontaneous immunization of close contacts. The article concludes by saying, "Although wild polioviruses types 1 and 3 have been more difficult to control than type 2, the experience in the Americas, Western Pacific, and Europe underscores the feasibility of global eradication of all wild poliovirus serotypes."

In the three years following the 1988 launch of the Global Polio Eradication Initiative, the number of reported polio cases decreased dramatically. This was followed by a slight increase, until renewed efforts reversed the upswing. In 1995, 120 countries had had no cases to report in three years, but these were in regions where economic conditions and public health were satisfactory, and where the governments themselves took on most of the cost and logistics of immunization.

As the focal point shifted toward poorer countries, it

became necessary to find new impetus and sources of funding. The WHO estimated that $100 million more would be needed annually until 2000, the target year in which the organization had considered eradication to be possible.

China introduced its first National Immunization Days in December 1993. Some thirty-six countries organized National Immunization Days in 1994; sixty-two countries in 1995; and by 1996 there were eighty-six countries organizing NIDs. In 1997, one-third of the world's children under five were vaccinated during the NIDs. Nevertheless, the WHO found that, in a few dozen countries, the immunization coverage rate of children under five was not budging. Eradicating the virus in a few countries where the social, economic, or political situation was particularly difficult was proving to be a lengthier and more arduous task than expected.

Bruce Aylward emphasizes that "[i]f everyone had started when the resolution was decided in 1988, I think we would have reached our objective. The immunization campaigns did not really begin until 1995 in Europe and 1996 in Africa. And the world has changed a lot. In 1988, there was no war in Afghanistan, in the Congo, or in Somalia. In many regions of the world the environment has become very complicated to work in."

It became clear that the objective of eradicating polio by 2000 could not be attained. The initiative has now set its sights on a polio-free world in 2005, which means the disappearance of cases of polio due to the wild virus after 2002.

———

New partners have joined the Global Polio Eradication Initiative. The Bill and Melinda Gates Foundation has donated $50 million, and De Beers, the diamond company, has contributed $2.7 million. On October 11, 1999, Aventis Pasteur announced that the company would donate 50 million doses of vaccine to be used in five African countries. Governments have provided aid, or donated more than they had initially committed. Australia has given $1.5 million for China; Canada, $4 million for Nigeria and $10 million for the Global Initiative in 2001; Italy, $1 million for India; Japan, $28.6 million for six countries; the Netherlands, $51 million; and Great Britain, $50 million. Celebrities and star athletes have become ambassadors for the cause: supermodel Claudia Schiffer and tennis star Martina Hingis; actors and actresses such as Roger Moore and Mia Farrow; and Ted Turner, founder of Cable News Network and president of the private United Nations Foundation.

Millions of children have been saved from disability. The lives of hundreds of thousands have been spared. Beyond the humanitarian benefits of this initiative, it makes economic sense for industrialized countries to provide the Global Polio Eradication Initiative with the funds it needs.

Researchers at the National Institutes of Health in Bethesda, Maryland, have evaluated the health care and physical therapy savings attributable to the eradication of polio and compared them to the cost of the eradication campaign. Basing their estimates on eradication in 2000, they considered that the benefits would outweigh the costs from 2007 onward and that total savings would amount to $13.6 million in 2040. Moving the eradication target date to 2005 simply postpones the potential savings. To this must be added $1.7 billion dollars per year in savings when vaccination is finally discontinued.

As long as even one case of polio exists anywhere in the world, no country can take the risk of stopping polio vaccination. If the virus were reintroduced into an unvaccinated population with no natural immunization acquired through

Table 11.2
*Donor Profiles for Contributions Received and Announced,
1985–2002*

Contributions (in millions of dollars)	Public Sector Partners	Development Banks	Private Sector Partners
>500	United States		Rotary International
250 to 500	United Kingdom		
100 to 249	Japan, Netherlands	World Bank	
50 to 99	Germany		Bill and Melinda Gates Foundation
25 to 49	Canada, Denmark		United Nations Foundation
5 to 24	Australia, Belgium, European Commission, Norway, UNICEF and WHO standard budgets	Inter-American Development Bank	Aventis Pasteur, FIIM
1 to 4	ECHO, Ireland, Italy, Luxemburg, Sweden, Switzerland		De Beers, Wyeth

Total Contributions: $2.2 billion.

Source: World Health Organization, September 2002.

exposure to the virus during childhood, the consequences would be disastrous. The Netherlands learned this painful lesson in 1992.

For fourteen years, not a single case had been reported in the Netherlands, when a virus from India infected the members of a congregation of an Orthodox Reformed Church, who are opposed to all vaccination, in the village of Streefkerk. Seventy-one individuals aged ten days to sixty-one years fell ill. Two died and fifty-nine were paralyzed. The government spent $10 million to vaccinate all those at risk to contain the epidemic.

To avoid such a large-scale catastrophe, industrialized countries spend large sums of money to maintain immunization coverage even when polio has been eradicated within their borders. In the United States, $230 million is spent annually on polio prevention.

In developing countries, the Global Polio Eradication Initiative has had immediate positive consequences in other areas of public health. In 2001, staff employed by the WHO for the polio campaign devoted 44 percent of its time to routine immunization and epidemiological surveillance for international personnel, and 22 percent for national personnel. UNICEF takes advantage of the immunization campaigns to administer Vitamin A to children. Vitamin A deficiency increases mortality rates due to various diseases by 20 percent and can cause blindness. Fifty countries distributed Vitamin A during the National Immunization Days in 1999. According to the WHO, this saved 242,000 lives.

National Immunization Days often provide the opportunity to reorganize public health systems in developing countries, helping to establish antennas within the communities and set up the logistical organization required for the cold chain. NIDs contribute to the development of what the WHO calls a "vaccination culture," which facilitates the administration of all vaccines. Between 1990 and 1994, immunization coverage against tuberculosis, diphtheria, tetanus, pertussis, and measles increased by one-third in Cambodia and doubled in Laos.

A WHO symposium held in December 1999 came to the conclusion, however, that such positive repercussions are not automatic. If NIDs are not planned carefully, they can clash with local health-care systems and weaken other programs. The WHO has drawn up a "Checklist and indicators for optimizing the impact of polio activities on EPI." A laminated card that sets out these guidelines is distributed throughout the world.

Despite so many successes, the international community is not sufficiently mobilized. In May 2001, Dr. Gro

Table 11.3
Breakdown of Projected Expenditures, 2003–2005

Immunization operations and activities	36%
Purchase of OPV	31%
AFP surveillance	16%
Mop-up campaigns, awareness, certification, confinement, strategy determination	17%

Total projected expenditures: $725 million.

Source: World Health Organization, September 2002.

Harlem Brundtland, director-general of the World Health Organization, sounded the alarm at an assembly of the organization. "The greatest threat to realizing the goal of polio eradication is the $400 million funding gap. Without the money, we cannot finish the job. We need sustained political commitment, too, with every political leader focused on the goal to keep polio eradication high on the political agenda."

Her call was heard, but in November 2002 the WHO announced that it was still $275 million short, $50 million of which was needed for the first six months of 2003.

The fight against polio became, in the middle of the twentieth century, the largest of all popular movements against disease. Millions of people contributed to the March of Dimes to care for polio victims and fund the discovery of a vaccine. In 1954, the Francis Field Trial to test the Salk vaccine was a success thanks to thousands of volunteers and hundreds of thousands of children, making it the largest medical experiment in history. Driven by the same momentum, the Global Polio Eradication Initiative has mustered the forces of the largest-ever international mobilization in times of peace.

It is remarkable that a decision made in Geneva—the outcome of politically balanced decisions, following the procedures and language that characterize large international assemblies—should meet with such enthusiasm in far-flung regions of the globe, in places that, socially and politically, could not be more unlike the shores of Lake Geneva. Like Archana Mudger of Uttar Pradesh, millions heard the appeal and stepped forward.

In nations with only the most rudimentary infrastructure, health authorities and volunteers do everything they can to make mothers aware of what is at stake and to reach as many children as possible.

In Burkina Faso, tribal chiefs hand down instructions that all children are to be brought to vaccination sites to receive their drops of OPV. After religious services, imams and priests announce when NIDs are to be held. Town criers call out to mothers in the markets. Vaccinators go from concession to concession, on foot, by bicycle or by scooter.

In India, famous actors make TV clips and religious communities hold prayer vigils where they exhort adults to vaccinate their children; volunteer organizations form processions of torch bearers and drummers wind their way through the streets on camels bedecked with banners; in the Himalayas the vaccines are borne by donkeys.

In industrialized countries, Rotary members continue to collect large amounts of money. Together with the WHO, UNICEF, and the CDC, they stubbornly knock on government doors to obtain the funding they need.

The momentum of such efforts cannot be sustained indefinitely. The only viable option at the beginning of the twenty-first century is rapid, total victory. Anything less will mean that the energy expended by so many people for over ten years will have been wasted.

12

The End

Game

Kenya and Sudan, November 2000 and India, January 2001

Lokichoggio, Kenya, Saturday, November 18, 2000. The UNICEF cold room is buzzing with activity. It has been set up in a tent at the camp the United Nations uses as its base for the Lifeline Sudan operation. From here, UNICEF and nongovernmental organizations provide assistance to some 5.4 million inhabitants of southern Sudan, amid the ravages of the African continent's oldest civil war.

UNICEF employees load large ice boxes filled with oral polio vaccines into trucks. The containers will be transferred to five airplanes, not far from the camp, which fly the United Nations colors. The planes are scheduled to leave the next morning for over eighty landing strips in southern Sudan.

Sudan, a country of 23 million inhabitants, is about one-quarter the size of the United States. It was the arena of armed conflicts from its independence in 1955 until 1972. Civil war broke out in 1983 and has not abated since. The southern part of the country is in conflict with the ruling powers in Khartoum, where a military dictatorship promulgating an Islamic government took over after a coup d'état in 1989. Nearly two million people have lost their lives, and more than twice as many have been displaced. The situation is complicated by the fact that the rebel zone is shared by many rival groups of militia.

Southern Sudan is one of the ten priority target areas identified by the WHO to bring the number of cases of poliomyelitis to zero. Five of these target areas are in countries where war has kept children from being immunized: Sudan, Angola, the Democratic Republic of the Congo, Somalia, and Afghanistan. The five other countries are considered "reservoirs" because they are characterized by a combination of high population density, poor sanitation, and very low immunization coverage: India, where over one half of all cases worldwide occur, Bangladesh, Ethiopia, Nigeria, and Pakistan. It is in these ten countries that the "end game," as the WHO calls it, is being played out—the home stretch in the race to eradicate polio. If the virus continues to circulate in just one outlying village, or just one overpopulated slum in just one of these countries, it can be spread by travelers to the entire world.

In the last decade of the twentieth century, polio epidemics broke out in many war-torn parts of the globe: in Chechnya in 1995 (150 cases); in Iraq after the Gulf War and then again in 1999 in the northern part of the country; in Albania in 1996, whence it spread to Kosovo and Greece; in Sudan; and, most seriously, in Angola in 1999. From March 1 to May 28, 1999, Angola suffered the worst polio epidemic ever seen in Africa. In and around the capital, Luanda, 1,093 cases were reported. More than 80 of them were fatal.

On November 19 and 20, 2000, new National Immunization Days were organized in southern Sudan. The dates were negotiated with the secessionist leaders and the authorities in Khartoum. Bombing ceased and the United Nations planes carrying vaccines were able to take off.

The vaccines airlifted from Lokichoggio were part of Aventis Pasteur's donation of 50 million doses of oral vaccine presented to the WHO on October 11, 1999. These vaccines are being supplied over a three-year period for the National Immunization Days in five war-torn African countries: Sudan, Angola, Liberia, Sierra Leone, and Somalia. This is an example of the effectiveness of partnerships that are forged within the framework of the Global Polio Eradication Initiative.

According to Michel Gréco, deputy CEO of sanofi-aventis, "This is how Aventis Pasteur is expressing its solidarity with the WHO in its fight to eradicate polio from the globe. We hope that our contribution will encourage all those involved in eradication to continue their efforts. If industry can make a donation, there is no reason why others can't do the same. For our donation to have a more dramatic impact, we have targeted five African countries who are in dire need of foreign help because they are being completely destroyed by war."

The partnership with the vaccine industry goes well beyond donations. The polio eradication campaign was launched in a context where a new kind of relationship has developed between international organizations and pharmaceutical laboratories. The campaign has given impetus to the change.

The fight against AIDS has also influenced this relationship. For more than 95 percent of people living with AIDS, the price of treatment is prohibitively high. As a result, today governments, international organizations, NGOs, and pharmaceutical laboratories are obliged to work together in order to establish different prices depending on the buyer country. They have also set up programs to facilitate access to care.

In the field of vaccines, the Global Alliance for Vaccines

and Immunization (GAVI) is a partnership in the true sense of the word. GAVI is unique. It is not a new organization, but an alliance whose purpose is to "increase children's access to vaccination in developing countries" through the joint efforts of international organizations, buyers and users of vaccines, manufacturers, NGOs, and the Bill and Melinda Gates Foundation. GAVI has created a fund to finance immunization in poor countries.

"One of the consequences of the effort required for the polio eradication campaign is that representatives of industry and international organizations have come to know one another better," says Robert Sebbag, executive vice president of communications at sanofi-aventis. "Partnership is essential for our work to be effective. The WHO cannot plan an immunization strategy if it does not ask industry how many doses of OPV and IPV it can provide by 2010. We in industry, on the other hand, need to know what to expect. If the WHO suddenly decided that OPV would be discontinued and replaced entirely by IPV, all the vaccine manufacturers in the world would not be able to produce enough vaccine. We must have an ongoing dialogue."

———

One of the planes that takes off from Lokichoggio flies over the Sudd Swamp between the Blue Nile and the White Nile. This vast expanse of shallow water is filled with reeds and river grass; it is hard to say where the land begins and where it ends. In times past, the Sudanese Nuer tribe roamed here on foot, carrying their children on their backs. The area, not easily accessible at the best of times and surrounded by pockets where the fighting continues, has reverted to its wild state.

The plane approaches Pabuong, a settlement of a few dozen huts. The pilot, formerly with the Ethiopian army, circles the landing strip several times to clear it of children and cattle before he lands. As soon as the two cases of vaccine are unloaded, he takes off for Nyal.

Many families from the other side of the Nile, where the fighting is especially violent, have taken refuge in the village of Nyal. In the event of an attack, it is easy to hide here, on one of the thousands of small islands in the swamp, where soldiers unfamiliar with the area stand no chance of finding their way around. There are hardly any men—just women, small children, and a few old people. The UN pilots, who are authorized to fly over only part of the region, spot troops of elephants from their planes. Even these great lumbering beasts take refuge here.

This is the first time UNICEF has conducted an operation of this type. On November 20, the vaccinators arrive with their ice boxes in flat-bottomed, propeller-driven airboats that are similar to the boats used to navigate the Florida Everglades. Their plan is to make a stop at every island in the area they have been assigned.

Stepping onto one of the islands, the volunteers use loudspeakers to announce their arrival. They go from hut to hut, drawing a cross on the wall as they leave to show which huts have been visited. In one hut, they find two soldiers from an unidentified militia. At the far end of the village, they come across a family of a dozen women and children, newly arrived after traveling for seven days in a flat bark to cross the Nile and the swamp.

When the vaccinators return to Nyal at the end of the day, few children have escaped the mopping-up operation. And the volunteers know that those who did not receive the three drops of OPV will probably be protected by contact with other children who were immunized.

In countries at war, the UN attempts to negotiate "Days of Tranquility" with all parties concerned, during which all fighting ceases so that vaccination can take place. Such days were organized in the Republic of the Congo and in Angola in 1999, 2000, and 2001.

Unfortunately, the ceasefire and the assurance of safe passage are not always enforced. For example, between July 5 and 10, 2001, the WHO synchronized the National Immunization Days held in Angola, the Congo, the Democratic Republic of the Congo, and Gabon. The WHO sought to increase the chances of reaching children displaced from one country to another. According to the British scientific journal *Nature*, 20 percent of the children in Angola were in zones where the UNITA (National Union of the Total Independence of Angola) rebels refused access to vaccinators. The WHO's efforts to encourage mothers to bring their children to the border might not have been adequate.

In addition to the five war-torn countries, the final phase of the Global Polio Eradication Initiative is concentrating its efforts on five reservoir countries: India, Bangladesh, Ethiopia, Nigeria, and Pakistan. In these states, the main obstacles to eradication have to do with reporting cases of polio and monitoring the circulation of the virus. High population density and poor sanitation facilitate the spread of the poliovirus. Largely inadequate health services cannot reach children who contract the disease.

In the mid-1990s, the campaign to eradicate polio made significant strides in India and other countries. The first mass vaccination using OPV was organized in the capital city of New Delhi in 1994, and the first NIDs were organized in 1995. In 1999, one billion OPV doses were administered during the NIDs. The number of polio cases made a spectacular drop, especially considering that the actual number of cases must have been much higher before a surveillance system was set up in 1997: 3,263 cases were reported in

1995; 4,316 were reported in 1998; 461 in 1999; and 250 in 2000.

In January 2001, a heavy padlock was hung on the Polio Room located in the overcrowded, noisy, and foul-smelling basement of the Kalawati Saran Children's Hospital in New Delhi. The hospital still occasionally receives patients with polio, but the children are sent to the general wards. In 2000, only three cases of poliomyelitic paralysis were reported in the capital, where six years previously the incidence of polio was one of the highest in the world.

The situation in India is one of sharp contrasts. The circulation of the wild poliovirus was stopped in 1998 in twelve of the thirty-two Indian states. In 2000, 85 percent of all cases (218 cases), were concentrated in the two poorest states, Bihar and Uttar Pradesh. The WHO and its partners are focusing their efforts on thirty-nine of Uttar Pradesh's districts and fifteen of Bihar's, where there are no fewer than 22 million children under five years of age

Gary Hlady is responsible for polio surveillance in India. He has been sent by the CDC to organize the National Polio Surveillance Project.

"In 1997, we hired and trained the first 59 doctors who took charge of poliomyelitis surveillance," he says. "Today we have some 200 doctors throughout the country. Most of them specialize in preventive medicine or public health. Two-thirds of them worked for the civil service and will return to their jobs when the program is completed. This is how we are training them for the future.

"The system we are establishing will be used to track other diseases, like measles and neonatal tetanus. We have already been asked to take action to stop other epidemics, such as outbreaks of measles."

Polio surveillance is the fourth pillar of the strategy of

the Global Polio Eradication Initiative, along with routine immunization, NIDs, and house-to-house mopping-up campaigns. Surveillance is based on recording cases of Acute Flaccid Paralysis.

"The aim of the surveillance network is to detect all cases of AFP," says Gary Hlady. "Each time a case occurs, the patient's stools are sent to one of the seven certified polio laboratories for analysis and virus detection."

"We have an extremely sure method to verify the reliability of the surveillance network. We know that in any country, independently of polio, at least one case of AFP due to other causes per 100,000 children occurs annually. If the annual number of reported cases of AFP not caused by polio is at least one per 100,000 children, we can deduce that any case of AFP caused by polio would be reported as well. In India, we reached the threshold of one per 100,000 nationwide in May 1998."

Setting up the network in the field required the dedication, patience, and sense of initiative of the doctors in charge of surveillance, who are referred to as surveillance medical officers. Dr. Kamal Chand Singhal is an SMO in Aligarh, a city of over one million people.

"The WHO had begun recording cases of AFP (Acute Flaccid Paralysis) in the Aligarh region in October 1997," says Dr. Singhal, "but when I arrived, on July 27, 1999, not a single case of polio (confirmed wild polio virus) had been reported since January 1999. One could have concluded that this was because of good vaccination activities, so there was no more polio. But actually it was because the Acute Flaccid Paralysis cases were not being reported. This showed poor Acute Flaccid Paralysis surveillance.

"I got in touch with the doctors at the medical centers and those practicing traditional medicine, and I called on journalists to keep both me and the other doctors informed. By December 31, 1999, I had identified 32 cases of confirmed polio (wild virus positive). Thus I could identify the pockets where the virus was circulating and where immunization efforts had to be focused. Today, Acute Flaccid Paralysis surveillance is efficient, because we have more than one case of non-polio AFP per every 100,000 children under the age of fifteen.

"The situation in these regions poses particular problems. For example, when I took the job there was no map of the city. It was impossible to locate epidemic outbreaks and organize door-to-door operations. So one of the first things that I did was to draw up a map, so that we could ensure 100 percent immunization coverage and work toward achieving the goal of polio eradication.

"Then I solved the problem of people who claimed that the Muslim community was opposed to vaccination. I called the leaders of the Muslim community together, and the Mufti quoted a verse of the Koran that says that the health of children is the sole responsibility of parents, and that they should make every effort to protect their children's health. So in fact there was no Muslim opposition. Public health workers had used this as a pretext not to do anything in the most difficult neighborhoods.

"Then there is the crime rate. After five in the evening, even the police refuse to go into certain neighborhoods. Kidnapping is widespread in this State, and this makes it difficult to move around."

The efforts made by Dr. Singhal, Shivam NGO, Gyatri Pariwar, the students of the Islamic School of Medicine, and all the volunteers have paid off. The SMOs recorded only a single case of polio in 2000, a child who was paralyzed in January.

13

The

Challenge of

Eradication

Spring 2003

As the year 2002 drew to a close, it became clear that the World Health Organization's goal of eradicating all cases of polio caused by the wild virus would not be reached. Not only did the virus continue to spread, but the number of polio cases was higher than in 2001. In addition, virologists were troubled by another concern: cases of vaccine-associated polio were reported years after immunization campaigns with the oral vaccine. Eradicating polio would be more complicated than what had been generally expected.

Worldwide, the successes of the polio campaign continued. On June 21, 2002, a meeting of the Regional Commission for Certification of Polio Eradication declared that polio had disappeared from the WHO European region, which included fifty-one countries and 870 million people. Cases of paralysis caused by imported viruses were reported in Bulgaria and Georgia in 2001, but no case of polio caused by a locally contracted virus had been observed for more than three years. The condition for certification had been met.

Europe was the third WHO region to be declared polio-free, following the Americas in 1994 and the Western Pacific in 2000.

In 2001, the global incidence of polio had continued to drop, with 483 cases reported, seven times fewer than in 2000. The virus was circulating in only ten countries on two continents. No type 2 wild virus has been isolated since 1999, and it is possible that type 2 has been eliminated across the globe. In 2002, the number of polio endemic countries fell to seven, but the number of cases was on the rise in Egypt, Nigeria, and especially India. Globally the number of cases had increased to 1,918.

In light of this paradoxical situation, while the prospects for eradication had improved overall, they had worsened in these three countries. For Bruce Aylward, coordinator of the Global Eradication Initiative, each of these three countries represents a special case, each with its own particular challenges, requiring an appropriate response. He explains:

> What is most disturbing in Egypt is that the cases are from different parts of the country. Genetically they are quite different, which means there is much more transmission than people have been recognizing. Numerous cases of polio have gone unreported. We collaborate with public health officials at the highest level to improve the reliability of the surveillance network. Four rounds of National Immunization Days (NIDs) were organized in 2003. Because there is so little polio in Egypt, and because of other factors, this should be able to eliminate the disease very fast.
>
> Cases in Nigeria are found in the northern part of this vast country. The pattern is not that of an epidemic

Table 13.1

Number of Cases of Polio in 2002, 2003, and 2004

Country	2002	2003	2004
Pakistan	90	103	23
India	1,600	225	34
Nigeria	202	355	476
Afghanistan	10	8	3
Benin*	0	2	6
Niger	3	40	19
Burkina Faso*	1	11	6
Central African Republic*	0	1	3
Cameroon*	0	2	1
Chad*	0	25	12
Ghana*	0	8	0
Togo*	0	1	0
Egypt	7	1	1
Lebanon*	0	1	0
Somalia	3	0	0
Zambia*	2	0	0
Sudan*	0	0	5
Guinea*	0	0	1
Mali*	0	0	2
Botswana*	0	0	1
Ivory Coast*	0	1	9
Total	1,918	784	602

* Virus imported from another country or under analysis.
Source: Data centralized by the World Health Organization as of August 24, 2004, and compared with 2002 and 2003 (confirmed infections due to wild virus).

(when the number of cases explodes because of the rapid spread of the virus), but more of an endemic one (a steady number of annual cases, similar to what occurred in many countries before the eradication campaign started). Immunization campaigns were not carried out as effectively in this region of the country. The increase we are seeing no doubt corresponds to a marked improvement in surveillance. There are not more cases; we are simply better at finding them. We believed that surveillance for the entire country was as good as in the south, where infrastructures are better, and believed that the drop in the number of cases was greater than it actually was.

Three local NIDs were organized in 2003 in the northern states of Nigeria. The WHO estimated that if these NIDs were well organized, the spread of the virus within the country could be stopped over the course of the year.

India is another country where the global eradication initiative faces its greatest hurdles: 85 percent of polio cases contracted in 2002 occurred in India, and three-quarters of these were in Uttar Pradesh, one of the country's poorest states.

According to Bruce Aylward, "Surveillance has been good for the last few years. What we are seeing is a massive epidemic of the type 1 virus, caused by multiple factors. In 2002, India cut back on the number of rounds of immunization and the rounds did not reach enough children. We saw that a substantial proportion of children has never been immunized, primarily in Muslim communities."

A study conducted by the WHO in western Uttar Pradesh revealed that in the Hindu community, 93 percent of children between the ages of six months and five years had received at least four doses of OPV and 7 percent had received from one to three doses. In the Muslim community, 77 percent of children in the same age group had received at least four doses, 19 percent from one to three doses, and 4 percent not a single dose.

A rumor spread among the Muslim community that the OPV drops the authorities were making such a fuss about, the drops that strangers were so anxious to deposit into the mouths of their children, even venturing into the slums where no one ever set foot, were actually intended to sterilize them. The rumor was that the privileged Hindu class wanted to keep the Muslim population from reproducing.

"With the program, we've heard these rumors in other areas of the world," says Bruce Aylward. "One of the dangers at this stage in India is that people are starting to say the problem is that the community will not accept the program. And now the most vulnerable, poor, marginalized community is being blamed for its own problem. In reality, things are much more complex than that. There is a certain degree of refusal of immunization, but it is not the fault of the community, which has never had health services brought to its door; nobody has cared about their children. These are not stupid people. They may be illiterate, but they are not stupid."

Bruce Aylward's opinion coincides with the viewpoint expressed by Anne-Marie Moulin, who believes it is time to "stop attributing people's resistance, refusal, or reticence about vaccination to their invincible backwardness."[1] Because immunization targets the individual, touches the body, and is essentially imposed by the authorities, it is a catalyzer for political and social tensions. When, in 1904, in Rio de Janeiro, the Brazilian government made the smallpox vaccine mandatory, the population's response was the *Rivolta da vacina*, an insurrection that was met with bloody repression. In the first half of the nineteenth century "variolization" (inoculating healthy subjects with pus from pox sores) had also prompted hostile reactions in Algeria and Egypt.

The difficulties encountered by the polio campaign in Uttar Pradesh echo a movement of resistance to the tetanus vaccine in Cameroon in the last years of the twentieth century. In order to prevent neonatal tetanus, which is often caused when an unsterilized instrument is used to sever the umbilical cord, the government of Cameroon made tetanus immunization obligatory for all women ages fourteen to forty-two. The northeastern part of the country was experiencing a period of political instability and, given the target population, the campaign was perceived as a massive sterilization program. Fears increased after the murder of a priest who had challenged the central government. Young girls stopped going to school, and clashes between the local population and the police brought the region to a state of near-siege.

In the Muslim neighborhoods in Uttar Pradesh, India, which are among the poorest urban slums in the world, the government health services never come to call and no one ever sees a nurse, much less a doctor. The last time health services came into this area, it was for a sterilization program in the mid-1970s. "The government in Uttar Pradesh and the other sectors need to get the Muslim community involved," says Bruce Aylward. "Not just in receiving the vaccine, but they need to take part in planning the National Immunization Days and deciding about financial allocations. We must overcome a century of distrust.

"In fact, many people don't get a chance to say 'no' because the vaccine is not offered to their children. Up to 10 percent of houses are not properly visited in high risk areas, in neighborhoods where people live packed together, with poor sanitation. This percentage is just too high."

Bruce Aylward is optimistic about the future; he believes the government in Uttar Pradesh knows "it cannot afford to be the country that prevents polio eradication" and is aware of the tremendous responsibility it would have, in the eyes of the rest of the world, if the global eradication campaign fails because of the failure in this state. Six series of NIDs were organized in 2003 in Uttar Pradesh, where more than two million children are born each year. The NIDs of February 2003, which targeted 150 million children, were the largest immunization campaign in history.

In India and globally, the eradication campaign has

reached a point of no return. The circulation of the virus has been stopped in most countries, and tens of millions of young children who have never been exposed to the virus have not acquired natural immunity. Bruce Aylward explains that "if we fail, we are not going to go back to a few thousand cases a year. There will be hundreds of thousands of cases again in five years and polio will have spread from India to anywhere in the world." Between 1999 and 2002, the WHO identified at least ten instances of the virus being imported to countries where polio had disappeared. In 2002, epidemic outbreaks developed in certain Indian states where polio had disappeared. The virus was imported from Uttar Pradesh.

The WHO estimates that an additional $100 million in international funding will be necessary to organize more immunization campaigns, because the objective of eliminating all cases of polio by the end of 2002 was not met. The Rotary International Board of Directors is convinced that "the greatest obstacle to victory is inadequate funding" and is following the WHO's call to raise $275 million by 2005 to bring the eradication campaign to a successful conclusion. The board decided to launch a one-year fundraising campaign. Rotary's objective was to raise $80 million in cash and pledges between July 1, 2002, and June 30, 2003, and on June 3, 2003, the Rotarians had already raised $88.5 million. The Bill and Melinda Gates Foundation committed an additional $25 million.

As eradication draws closer, meetings, symposia, and scientific articles discuss the immunization strategy to be pursued when polio is finally eradicated everywhere. Even after eradication, the virus will continue to circulate. The wild poliovirus can be transmitted for some time before being detected, since it leads to symptoms in only one in two hundred infected individuals.

The most difficult task, paradoxically, may turn out to be eliminating the virus contained in the oral polio vaccine. One of the main advantages of the OPV is that it allows the live attenuated virus to be transmitted from person to person, which automatically immunizes the people who are in contact with an immunized child. The virus, however, mutates as it reproduces and, over time, it may at times become as virulent as the wild poliovirus. Taking into consideration vaccinated individuals and their families, it has long been estimated that OPV vaccination results in approximately one case of paralysis for every 750,000 to one million doses administered. According to the WHO, this figure is actually one case for every 2.5 million doses.

The virus contained in the vaccine was generally believed to disappear after a few months. An article published in 2000 in a special issue of the *Bulletin of the WHO* put forward three hypotheses. First, that the virus transmitted by OPV probably circulates in the population for a limited amount of time, three months at the most according to data available at the time. Second, "poliomyelitis outbreaks are invariably due to wild type strains rather than vaccine-derived strains, suggesting that the vaccine-derived poliovirus may be less transmittable than wild type strains." Third, when the virus combines with other enteroviruses, in an exchange of genetic material from viruses in the same family as the poliovirus, such recombinants have low virulence and "are unlikely to pose a threat to the eradication program."

Cases of polio declared in 2000 and 2001 in the Dominican Republic and Haiti, which together form the island of Hispaniola, revealed that reality is not so simple. From July 2000 to July 2001, twenty-one cases of polio were confirmed in these two countries, including two fatal cases, even though the Americas had been certified polio-free in 1994.

Genetic analysis of the viruses found in the patients' stools showed that the viruses originated from a single dose of OPV administered in late 1998 or early 1999. This suggested that vaccine-derived virus may circulate at least eighteen months in a community before it reverts to pathogenicity, which is much longer than anyone had thought up to that point.

Genetic analysis also disproved another certainty: all the analyzed viruses came from a recombinant of the vaccine strain and an enterovirus. According to the authors of an article published in April 2002 in *Science*, "At least four different enteroviruses" had recombined with the type 1 virus from the vaccine. Contrary to expectations, this recombination had produced viruses that had recovered the capacity to cause severe paralytic disease and the capacity for extensive person-to-person transmission.

With eradication approaching and the urgent need to determine the amount of time OPV-derived poliovirus can circulate, in recent years researchers have been studying stool samples that were taken in the past from patients with vaccine-associated paralysis.

Genetic analysis was performed on viruses found in samples taken from thirty-two people in Egypt who were victims of vaccine-associated polio from 1988 to 1993. The OPV-derived virus had begun circulating in approximately 1982; it had therefore spread among the population for five years before recovering neurovirulence. This virus was then transmitted for five more years before immunization campaigns eliminated it. The cases of paralysis corresponded to ten chains of transmission.

The Egyptian cases were caused by a type 2 OPV-derived virus; type 2 wild poliovirus had stopped circulating in Egypt in 1979. These cases prefigured the scenario the WHO is trying to prepare for with regard to the three viral types. When wild type 1 and 3 strains are eliminated, just as type

2 may already be eliminated today worldwide, any outbreak of polio will be due to OPV-derived viruses.

In Egypt, as in the Dominican Republic and Haiti, it was possible for the virus to be transmitted for years because of low vaccination coverage. In a community with high coverage, OPV-derived virus is unable to find a continuous chain of susceptible individuals to infect and sustain its transmission. These countries are characterized by a double handicap: poor hygiene and low vaccination coverage.

According to the Centers for Disease Control, "The finding that vaccine-derived poliovirus may circulate under suitable conditions presents an additional challenge to efforts to eradicate polio worldwide."[2] Steve Cochi of the CDC says: "This discovery will not affect eradicating the last case of polio caused by wild poliovirus, but it will impact developing the proper end-game strategies to prevent similar circulating vaccine-derived poliovirus outbreaks from occurring in the post-eradication era."[3] As the WHO noted, these cases underline how difficult it is to maintain polio surveillance and immunization in developing countries once the disease has been declared eradicated in a given region.

Another area of concern for the post-eradication era is the issue of long-term shedding: immunodeficient individuals may be unable to eliminate the virus they ingested with OPV and may disseminate it for many years after being vaccinated.

An article published in 1997 describes an immunodeficient patient in the United States who harbored the virus for seven years, during which time the vaccine-derived virus mutated and reverted to neurovirulence. He received the OPV in 1974 and was diagnosed with polio in July 1981. In Germany, an immunodeficient child suffered paralysis three years after vaccination and continued to shed the virus for five and one-half years. In another patient, the virus persisted for nearly ten years. In Great Britain, an immunodeficient individual who showed no sign of illness shed the virus for up to fifteen years.

Although these examples are extreme and very rare, the vaccine-derived virus has been found in other patients for one, two, or three years. People who are immunodeficient due to a hereditary disease, AIDS, or treatment with immune suppressants may disseminate the virus in a community years after being immunized or infected by another person.

Today we know that the OPV-derived virus will continue to circulate for months or even years after the last case of polio. The worst-case scenario might be an immunodeficient individual who sheds the virus years after receiving the vaccine; this virus would then be transmitted for years before reverting to neurovirulence and being detected. Stopping immunization as soon as polio is declared officially eradicated by the WHO, three years after the last case due to wild poliovirus, could make people everywhere run a risk.

Donald Henderson, who directed the global campaign to eradicate smallpox and in 2003 advised President George W. Bush on bioterrorism issues, has for years been critical of the way in which the WHO eradication campaign has been organized. He is against stopping polio immunization: "It is important to bear in mind that the Assembly's commitment was to the eradication of polio, not the eradication of polio vaccine," he said. "These are two quite different goals and should not be confused."[4]

For Bruce Aylward, the risk is minimal and any eventual epidemics would be perfectly controllable: "The risk of vaccine-associated paralysis (VAP) is one out of 2.5 million doses of OPV given, which represents 250 to 500 cases per year. The risk of epidemics due to the vaccine, such as in Haiti, is smaller, since there have been twenty-nine cases in three years. Among immunocompromised individuals who carry the virus, nineteen have been identified since 1963, and only four of them continue to shed the virus. These cases are extremely rare. If you ask, 'Do we really want to continue using a vaccine that will cause paralysis, due to these very rare vaccine-derived epidemic outbreaks years later, and due to immunocompromised carriers of the virus?' the answer is generally negative."

The risk of epidemics due to viruses derived from vaccine strains will grow smaller over time to be almost nil four years after stopping OPV immunization.

The ultimate goal of polio eradication is to one day stop all polio immunization. But, until then, which vaccines should be given, and when? To date the WHO has not drawn up any recommendations on whether or not to continue immunization after certification of eradication. Regardless of the recommendations, each country will be free to determine its own health policy. The choice will not be the same in industrialized countries, where the polio vaccine is included in vaccine combinations and is not a burden on health-care costs, as in developing countries, where polio immunization is essentially ensured through mass campaigns and health-care budgets are very limited. In any event, national governments will have to work together, because stopping immunization cannot be accomplished by haphazard methods.

The decision to switch from OPV to IPV in certain countries, or to discontinue all immunization, will be, above all, a political decision. The question is whether policy makers will decide on a vaccine that is more expensive and must be administered by health-care personnel, to deal with a minor risk, after having eliminated the disease using an inexpensive vaccine that is mostly administered by volunteers.

The WHO created a Technical Consultative Group on the Global Eradication of Poliomyelitis, in charge of developing proposals to submit to the annual General Assembly, which is made up of representatives of member countries. The group recommended the following approach in the event of identification of vaccine-derived cases of polio:

- Two cases: mop-up campaigns in the region.
- One case: if when compared to the virus used in the vaccine, genetic drift is greater than 1 percent and there is recombination with another enterovirus (indicators of an epidemic risk), organize mop-up campaigns; if genetic drift is less than 1 percent, conduct an epidemiological study and organize mop-up campaigns if vaccine coverage is inadequate.

The Technical Group is preparing a field study to evaluate the feasibility of IPV immunization in developing countries, to replace OPV. Two projects should be set up to last five years.

———

The WHO also looked at another risk: after immunization programs have been stopped, there is a possibility that virus stored in laboratories might be inadvertently or deliberately released. This is not a far-fetched scenario: the last person to die of smallpox was infected when the virus escaped from a laboratory in Birmingham (United Kingdom) in 1978.

In February 2003, the committee of WHO experts on biological standardization issued recommendations for manufacturers of the injectable vaccine concerning the containment of virulent strains used to make the vaccine. Each country must set up special national groups to identify all the laboratories that are likely to have the virus; these laboratories will be asked to destroy their stock, to apply stricter safety measures (known as BSL-3), or to transfer their samples to WHO-approved stockpiles.

The WHO acknowledges that "it is impossible to guarantee that all laboratories will be identified" since stool samples or throat swab specimens may contain undetected virus. However, this plan "considerably reduces the risk of an accidental reintroduction of a wild poliovirus from a laboratory."

Discussions are also underway on the type and quantity of vaccine stockpiles to build up in the coming years to stop epidemics, after immunization has been discontinued, and, in the long term, to deal with a possible inadvertent or deliberate reintroduction of the poliovirus. The Technical Consultative Group recommends stockpiling monovalent OPV vaccines, i.e., containing the live attenuated virus of a single viral type, in order to avoid needlessly introducing the other two viral types for which immunization is not required.

The idea that polio could be used as a bioterrorist threat is hardly worth considering, since the virus paralyzes only one of every two hundred people it infects. Moreover, bioterrorism itself may be less of a news item by the time eradication has been declared, and the supposed threats or political reasons behind such threats may have disappeared by then.

Each in its own way, the smallpox and polio vaccines occupy a special place in the history of medicine. Variolization was the first type of immunization in the

The First Artificial Microbe

Right up to its eradication, polio will be associated with innovative discoveries. On July 11, 2002, a team of U.S. researchers announced that it had created a synthetic version of the poliovirus. Their findings were published in *Sciencexpress,* the online edition of the journal *Science.* The team had succeeded in creating a 100 percent artificial microbe.

Using the genetic map of the poliovirus, established years ago, and chemicals found routinely in laboratories worldwide, the team armed itself with patience as it aligned 7,741 bases to piece together synthetic poliovirus DNA. An enzyme was used to transcribe it into viral RNA, which functioned like real viral RNA and made proteins, ultimately forming infectious poliovirus.

Once global polio eradication has been achieved, the world will not be rid of a polio threat if unscrupulous scientists decide to synthesize the poliovirus. According to Dr. Alain Goudeau of the Bretonneau Teaching Hospital in Tours, France, this threat is insignificant compared to many others that he considers much more terrifying. "With the tools at our disposal today, we can envision some pretty horrible scenarios. For example, imagine that it is possible to graft components of the AIDS virus onto the influenza virus," he says (*Le Monde,* July 15, 2002). The WHO estimates that if used as a biological weapon, the poliovirus represents a small risk for public health, but that ending all polio vaccination could modify the evaluation of such a risk (*"Potentiel du poliovirus comme arme biologique,"* December 2001).

world, centuries before Louis Pasteur coined the term "vaccine." No peace-time cause has ever led to such a strong popular mobilization as the fight against polio, and no medical breakthrough has ever been as acclaimed as the first polio vaccine.

Thanks to the smallpox vaccine, human endeavor successfully eradicated an infectious disease for the first time in history. Will polio become the second such disease?

Notes

1 The Last Victims

1. Genetic analysis of the virus responsible for a case of polio identified on September 17, 2002, revealed that this virus had been imported from Nigeria.

2 A Lifetime Burden

1. *L'interactif*, no. 2, June 1998 (*Handicap International* and *Action Nord Sud* newsletter).

3 A Virus with a Long History

1. John R. Paul, *A History of Poliomyelitis* (New Haven and London: Yale University Press, 1971), p. 15.

4 The People versus Polio

1. Paul, *A History of Poliomyelitis*, pp. 190–196.
2. Christopher J. Rutty, "'Do Something . . . Do Anything!': Poliomyelitis in Canada, 1927–1962" (Ph.D. diss., University of Toronto, Department of History, 1995). See also Mr. Rutty's website, www.healthheritageresearch.com.
3. Jane S. Smith, *Patenting the Sun: Polio and the Salk Vaccine* (New York: William Morrow, 1990). This and subsequent chapters owe a great deal to Ms. Smith's excellent book.
4. Ibid., p. 51.
5. Ibid., p. 50.
6. Ibid., pp. 50–89 (through the end of this chapter).

6 Coming Along at the Right Time: Jonas Salk

1. Paul, *A History of Poliomyelitis*, pp. 257–260.
2. Ibid., pp. 233–235.

3. Smith, *Patenting the Sun*, p. 126.
4. Ibid., p. 125.
5. Ibid., p. 120.
6. Robert D. Defries, *The First Forty Years (1914–1955): Connaught Medical Research Laboratories* (Toronto: University of Toronto Press, 1968), p. 281.
7. Smith, *Patenting the Sun*, p. 127.
8. John A. Beale, "The Development of IPV," in *Vaccinia, Vaccination and Vaccinology: Jenner, Pasteur, and Their Successors*, ed. S. Plotkin and B. Fantini (Paris: Editions Elsevier, 1996), p. 221.
9. Roger Vaughan, *Listen to the Music: The Life of Hilary Koprowski* (New York: Springer, 2000), p. 48.
10. Smith, *Patenting the Sun*, p. 216.
11. Ibid., p. 199.

7   Behind the Scenes

1. *Time*, March 29, 1954, p. 60. Canadian edition.
2. Rutty, "Poliomyelitis in Canada," p. 296.
3. Quotations from Frank Shimada, employed by the Connaught Laboratories from 1949 to 1988, are taken from an interview conducted by Mary Shaffer in July 2000 in Toronto.
4. Rutty, "Poliomyelitis in Canada," p. 304.
5. Smith, *Patenting the Sun*, p. 236.
6. Defries, *The First Forty Years*, pp. 239–241, 271.
7. Ibid., p. 272.
8. Paul A. Bator, with A. Rhodes, *Within Reach of Everyone: A History of the University of Toronto School of Hygiene and the Connaught Laboratories*, vol. 1, *1927 to 1955* (The Canadian Public Health Association, 1990), p. 176.
9. Rutty, "Poliomyelitis in Canada," pp. 299–300.
10. Paul A. Bator, *Within Reach of Everyone: A History of the University of Toronto School of Hygiene and Connaught Laboratories Limited*, vol. 2, *1955 to 1975* (The Canadian Public Health Association, 1995), p. 93.
11. Defries, *The First Forty Years*, pp. 272–273.
12. Rutty, "Poliomyelitis in Canada," p. 309.
13. Bator, *Within Reach of Everyone*, 1:175–176.
14. Rutty, "Poliomyelitis in Canada," p. 315.
15. Smith, *Patenting the Sun*, p. 251.
16. Rutty, "Poliomyelitis in Canada," p. 195.

8   The Largest Medical Experiment in History

1. Smith, *Patenting the Sun*, p. 233.
2. Ibid., pp. 256–258.

3. Richard Carter, *The Gentle Legions* (New York: Doubleday, 1961), p. 133.
4. "Conquering the dreaded crippler, polio," The *Detroit News* web site: Rearview Mirror. http://detnews.com.
5. Smith, *Patenting the Sun*, p. 322.
6. Paul, *A History of Poliomyelitis*, pp. 432–433.
7. Ibid., pp. 436–438.
8. Defries, *The First Forty Years*, p. 280.

9   *The Race for an Oral Vaccine*

1. Hilary Koprowski, "Histoire alternative du vaccine oral," in *L'aventure de la vaccination*, under the direction of Anne-Marie Moulin (Paris: Fayard, 1996).
2. Vaughan, *Listen to the Music*, p. 51.
3. Ibid., pp. 51–56.
4. Bernard Seytre, *Sida: les secrets d'une polémique* (Paris: PUF, 1993); Bernard Seytre, *Histoire de la recherche sur le sida* (Paris: PUF, 1995).
5. Mentioned by John Paul, *A History of Poliomyelitis*.
6. Mentioned by John Paul, *A History of Poliomyelitis*.
7. Vaughan, *Listen to the Music*, p. 75.
8. Saul Benison, *Tom Rivers: Reflections on a Life in Medicine and Science* (Cambridge, MA: MIT Press, 1968), p. 152.
9. M. P. Chumakov et al., *Some Results of the Work on Mass Immunization in the Soviet Union with Live Poliovirus Vaccine Prepared from Sabin Strains* (World Health Organization, 1961).
10. Charles Mérieux, *Virus Passion* (Paris: Editions Robert Laffont, 1997).

10   *Revolution in the Production of Vaccines*

1. Mérieux, *Virus Passion*, 1997.
2. Japanese scientists speaking Esperanto coined the term "vero," a combination of *verda* and *reno* (green kidney).

11   *Polio: Programmed for Defeat*

1. Donald A. Hendersen, "Eradication: Lessons from the Past," *Morbidity and Mortality Weekly Report* 48, supplement, December 31, 1999 (Centers for Disease Control and Prevention).

13   *The Challenge of Eradication*

1. Anne-Marie Moulin, "L'hypothèse vaccinale: Pour une approche critique et anthropologique d'un phénomène historique." *Historia Ciência Saude Manguinhos*, 2003.

2. *Morbidity and Mortality Weekly Report* (Centers for Disease Control and Prevention), January 26, 2001.
3. Proceedings of the Symposium "No Room for Complacency" held in Ottawa, Canada, March 7–8, 2001.
4. *Immunization Focus*, quarterly publication of GAVI (Global Alliance for Vaccines and Immunization), December 2002, p. 6.

References

"Acute Flaccid Paralysis Associated with Circulating Vaccine-Derived Poliovirus, Philippines, 2001." *MMWR* 50, no. 40 (October 12, 2001).

Alexander, J. P., et al. "Duration of Poliovirus Excretion and Its Implications for Acute Flaccid Paralysis Surveillance: A Review of the Literature." *Journal of Infectious Diseases* 175, Suppl. 1 (1997): S176–S182.

"Apparent Global Interruption of Wild Poliovirus Type 2 Transmission." *MMWR* 50, no. 12 (March 30, 2001).

Bart, K. J., J. Foulds, and P. Patriarca. "Global Eradication of Poliomyelitis: Benefit-Cost Analysis." *Bulletin of the World Health Organization* 74, no. 1 (1996): 35–45.

Bator, Paul A. *Within Reach of Everyone. A History of the University of Toronto School of Hygiene and the Connaught Laboratories*, vol. 1 *(1927 to 1955)* and vol. 2, with Andrew J. Rhodes *(1955–1975)*. The Canadian Public Health Association, 1990 and 1995.

Beale, John A. "The Development of IPV." In *Vaccinia, Vaccination and Vaccinology: Jenner, Pasteur and Their Successors*, edited by S. Plotkin and B. Fantini. Paris: Elsevier, 1996.

Bellmunt, A., et al. "Evolution of Poliovirus Type I during 5.5 Years of Prolonged Enteral Replication in an Immunodeficient Patient." *Virology* 265 (1999): 178–184.

Benison, Saul. "International Medical Cooperation: Dr. Albert Sabin, Live Poliovirus Vaccine and the Soviets." *Bulletin of the History of Medicine* 56 (1982): 460–483.

Benison, Saul. *Tom Rivers: Reflections on a Life in Medicine and Science*. Cambridge, MA: MIT Press, 1968.

Berry, N., C. Davis, A. Jenkins, D. Wood, P. Minor, G. Schild, M. Bottiger, H. Holmes, and N. Almond. "Vaccine Safety: Analysis of Oral Polio Vaccine CHAT Stocks." *Nature* 410 (2001): 1046.

Blancou, P., J. P. Vartanian, C. Christopherson, N. Chenciner, C. Basilico, S. Kwok, and S. Wain-Hobson. "Polio Vaccine Samples Not Linked to AIDS." *Nature* 410 (2001): 1045.

Bodian, D., et al. "Differentiation of Types of Poliomyelitis Viruses." *American Journal Hygiene* 49 (1949): 234–245.

Carter, Richard. *The Gentle Legions*. New York: Doubleday, 1961.

Cello, J., et al. "Chemical Synthesis of Poliovirus cDNA." Sciencexpress, www.sciencexpress.org, July 11, 2002.

Chumakov, Mikhail et al. "Some Results of the Work on Mass Immunization in the Soviet Union with Live Poliovirus Vaccine Prepared from Sabin Strains." *Bulletin of the World Health Organization* 25 (1961): 79–91.

"Circulation of a Type 2 Vaccine-Derived Poliovirus, Egypt, 1952–1993." *MMWR* 50, no. 3 (January 26, 2001).

Clarke, Tom. "WHO Vaccinates 16 Million." *Nature Scienceupdate*, July 13, 2001.

"Confinement des Stocks de Poliovirus Sauvage." Geneva: World Health Organization, January 2002.

"Conquering the Dreaded Crippler, Polio," http://detnews.com. *Detroit News* website: Rearview Mirror.

Dalakas, M. C., et al. "Late Post-poliomyelitis Muscular Atrophy: Clinical, Virologic, and Immunologic Studies." *Reviews of Infectious Diseases* 6, Suppl. 2 (1984): S562–S567.

Defries, Robert D. *The First Forty Years, 1914–1955: Connaught Medical Research Laboratories, University of Toronto*. Toronto: University of Toronto Press, 1968.

Enders, J. F., et al. "Cultivation of the Lansing Strain of Poliomyelitis Virus in Cultures of Various Human Embryonic Tissues." *Science* 109 (1949): 85–87.

"Eradication of Poliomyelitis." Report by the World Health Organization Secretariat, Geneva, November 21, 2002.

Fondation Marcel Mérieux, à Lyon depuis 1897. Lyon: Marcel Mérieux Foundation.

Heim, A. "Prolonged Excretion of Vaccine-Derived Poliovirus in Immunodeficient Patients." *Recent Research and Development in Virology* 3 (2001): 395–407.

Henderson, Donald A. "Eradication: Lessons from the Past." *MMWR* 48, Suppl. (December 31, 1999).

Henderson, Donald A. "Lessons from the Eradication Campaigns." *Vaccine* 17 (1999): S53–S55.

Horstmann, D. M. "Poliomyelitis: Severity and Type of Disease in Different Age Groups." *Annals of New York Academy of Sciences* 61 (1955): 956–967.

Immunization Focus, a quarterly publication of the Global Alliance for Vaccines and Immunization (GAVI), December 2002.

Interactif, no. 2, June 1998 (newsletter published by "Handicap International" and the "Action Nord Sud" programs).

The Jordan Report 2000, Accelerated Development of Vaccines, NIH, USA.

Kew, Olen, et al. "Outbreak of Poliomyelitis in Hispaniola Associated with Circulating Type 1 Vaccine-Derived Poliovirus." *Science* 296 (2002): 356–359.

Koprowski, Hilary. "Histoire alternative du vaccine oral." In *L'aventure de la vaccination*, under the direction of Anne-Marie Moulin. Paris: Fayard, 1996.

Korber, B., M. Muldoon, J. Theiler, F. Gao, R. Gupta, A. Lapedes, B. H. Hahn, S. Wolinsky, and T. Bhattacharya. "Timing the Ancestor of the HIV-1 Pandemic Strains." *Science* 288 (2000): 1789–1796.

Louis, Cyrile. *Jonas Salk, victoire sur la polio.* Lyon: Pasteur Mérieux MSD, 1996.

Mérieux, Charles. *Virus Passion.* Paris: Editions Robert Laffont, 1997.

Minor, P. "Characteristics of Poliovirus Strains from Long-Term Excretors with Primary Immunodeficiencies." *Developmental Biology* (Basel) 105 (2001): 75–80.

Moulin, Anne-Marie. *Le dernier langage de la médecine.* Paris: Presses Universitaires de France, 1991.

Moulin, Anne-Marie. "L'hypothèse vaccinale: Pour une approche critique et anthropologique d'un phénomène historique." *Historia Ciência Saude Manguinhos*, 2003.

"New Polio Vaccines for the Post-eradication Era." Geneva: World Health Organization, 2000.

"No Room for Complacency," symposium proceedings, March 7–8, 2001, Ottawa.

Oostvogel, P. M., et al. "Poliomyelitis Outbreak in an Unvaccinated Community in the Netherlands, 1992–93." *Lancet* 344 (1994): 665–670.

"Outbreak of Poliomyelitis: Dominican Republic and Haiti, 2000." *MMWR* 49, no. 48, 1094 (December 8, 2000).

"Paralytic Poliomyelitis: United States, 1980–1994." *MMWR* 46, no. 4 (January 31, 1997).

Paul, John R. *A History of Poliomyelitis.* New Haven, CT: Yale University Press, 1971.

"Perspectives from the Dracunculiasis Eradication Programme." *MMWR* 48, Suppl. (December 31, 1999).

Plotkin, Stanley, and Edward A. Mortimer. *Vaccines.* 2d ed. Philadelphia, PA: W. B. Saunders Company, 1994.

Poinar, Hendrik, Melanie Kuch, and Svante Pääbo. "Molecular Analyses of Oral Polio Vaccine Samples." *Science* 292 (2001): 743–744. Published on-line April 25, 2001.

"*Polio, le commencement de la fin.*" Geneva: World Health Organization, 1998.

"*Politique de vaccination antipoliomyélitique de post-éradication.*" Geneva: World Health Organization, January 2002.

"Progress toward Poliomyelitis and Dracunculiasis Eradication: Sudan, 1999–2000." *MMWR* 50, no. 14 (April 13, 2001).

"Prolonged Poliovirus Excretion in an Immunodeficient Person with Vaccine-Associated Paralytic Poliomyelitis." *MMWR* 46, no. 28 (July 18, 1997): 641–643.

Rambaut, A., D. Robertson, O. G. Pybus, M. Peeters, and E. C. Holmes.

"Human Immunodeficiency Virus: Phylogeny and the Origin of HIV-1." *Nature* 410 (2001): 1047.

Relevé épidémiologique hebdomadaire. Geneva: World Health Organization.

Report of the Sixth Meeting of the Global Technical Consultative Group for Poliomyelitis Eradication. Geneva: World Health Organization, May 7–10, 2001.

Report of the Interim Meeting of the Technical Consultative Group on the Global Eradication of Poliomyelitis. Geneva: World Health Organization, November 13–14, 2002.

Rutty, Christopher J. "'Do Something! . . . Do Anything!' Poliomyelitis in Canada, 1927–1962." Ph.D. thesis, University of Toronto Department of History, 1995. See also Christopher Rutty's website: www.healthheritageresearch.com

Sabin, A. "Oral Poliovirus Vaccine: History of Its Development and Use and Current Challenge to Eliminate Poliomyelitis from the World." *Journal of Infectious Diseases* 151, no. 3 (1985).

Seytre, Bernard. *Histoire de la Recherche sur le Sida.* Paris: Presses Universitaires de France, 1995.

Seytre, Bernard. *Sida: les secrets d'une polémique.* Paris: Presses Universitaires de France, 1993.

Smith, Jane S. *Patenting the Sun: Polio and the Salk Vaccine.* New York: William Morrow, 1990.

"Special Theme: Polio Eradication." *Bulletin of the World Health Organization* 78, no. 3 (2000).

Sykes, Keith. "Mechanical Ventilation Goes Full Circle." On-line newsletter of the World Federation of Societies of Anesthesiologists, vol. 2, no. 1 (1998).

Vaccinia, Vaccination, Vaccinology, under the direction of S. Plotkin and B. Fantini. Paris: Elsevier, 1996.

Vaughan, Richard. *Listen to the Music: The Life of Hilary Koprowski.* New York: Springer, 2000.

Vitoux, Pierre. *La lutte contre la polio.* Paris: Nouvelles et Impressions, 1968.

Weiss, Robin A. "Polio Vaccines Exonerated." *Nature* 410 (2001): 1035.

Wood, D. J., R. W. Sutter, and W. R. Dowdle. "Stopping Poliovirus Vaccination after Eradication: Issues and Challenges." *Bulletin of the World Health Organization* 78, no. 3 (2002): 347–357.

World Health Organization press releases and fact sheets.

Internet sites:

http://www.post-polio.org
http://www.polioeradication.org
http://www.polio.info
http://www.rotary.org/foundation/polioplus/

Index

About the Authors

Bernard Seytre is a scientific journalist. His other works include: *Sida: les secrets d'une polémique* (Paris: Presses Universitaires de France [PUF], 1993); *Histoire de la Recherche sur le Sida* (PUF, 1995); and entries in *Dictionnaire d'histoire et philosophie des sciences* (PUF, 1999) and *Dictionnaire de la pensée médicale* (PUF, 2004).

Mary Shaffer is a Paris-based journalist and translator. She is the coauthor of *American Lawyers and Their Communities: Ethics in the Legal Profession* (University of Notre Dame Press, 1991).